The People's Repertory

2/26/04 at visit
to Dr Margo Roman

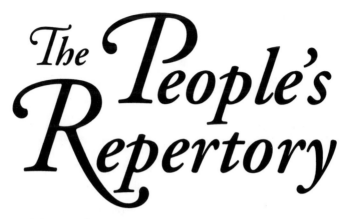

The People's Repertory

Your Guide to Safe, Effective Homeopathic Remedies

Luc De Schepper

M.D., Ph.D., C.Hom., D.I.Hom., Lic.Ac.

Full of Life Publishing • Santa Fe, NM

Disclaimer

This book is intended as an adjunct to, not substitute for, professional medical treatment. It is intended to assist readers in treating conditions which are not serious and which would be resolved in any case within a few days; or to support the patient while awaiting emergency medical treatment. The author and publisher are not responsible for any loss, damage or injury caused, or alleged to be caused, by the information contained in this book or for the misuse of the information. This book is in no way intended as a substitute for professional medical care.

Copyright © 1998 Luc De Schepper
ISBN 0-942-501-09-8
Full of Life Publishing
PO Box 31025
Santa Fe, NM 87594

Front cover: *antique mortar and pestle used to prepare homeopathic remedies and a collection of turn-of-the-century remedy bottles, including China (Cinchona), the first homeopathic remedy proved by Hahnemann.*

Cover photo credit: *Yolanda De Schepper*

Editorial and design: *Begabati Lennihan*

Illustrations: *Robert Rosa*

Proofreading: *Cat Weeks*

Contents

Dedication

To my beloved patients and staff in my New Jersey practice, for all the love I received from them, for all that I learned from them, and to show them that they will always be in my heart.

Introduction

Miracles and healing? They start with correcting the slightest imbalance in your body. Who is in a better position than you to respond to subtle emotional and physical changes in your own body? Your quest for health and longevity, a primary concern for all of us, starts with the help of this book.

When it comes to suffering, the division between allopathy (Western medicine) or homeo—pathy is of no importance. There are only patients who want relief from their suffering. It is for these people that this small book is intended. When a "classical" Western treatment is insufficient, or when patients simply want to be part of their healing process and add an excellent means of first aid to their armory, *The People's Repertory* can be a good source of information.

This manual does not pretend in any way to substitute for the family doctor or primary care physician (see Part One). No book can replace a physician's care. The reader of this book must realize the importance of an exact diagnosis which often does not fall within the layperson's domain. For this reason, this book covers acute, self-limiting conditions, to guide you while you are waiting for a further diagnosis and treatment from your physician. Having been in practice for the past 27 years, I know how valuable a simple book for the public can be. It will save time and money and it will prepare the way for further intervention by the physician, if necessary.

The limitations of this manual therefore explained, its necessity is obvious. There are many daily occurrences—physical, mental and emotional—which seem to be "not important enough" to call our physician for. Yet many of these so-called "innocent" acute events can often lead to chronic conditions. We must not underestimate the longterm effects of unresolved acute events on our health, acting like a slow leak from a tiny prick in the well-inflated balloon of our vital energy.

Of course, in addition to taking the appropriate remedy, other common sense measures should always be followed. These include rest, dietary changes in case of gastrointestinal illness, and a phone call to your partner on your health care team—your physician! This booklet does not authorize you to "impersonate a physician," distributing these magic little pellets to anyone you come in contact with. Besides small accidents and conditions for which you usually treat yourself (scrapes, bruises, minor burns, insect bites, etc.), this manual will also help you to perform first aid on your way to the doctor or the hospital.

PART ONE

Taking the Remedies: Frequently-Asked Questions

- ❖ *What is homeopathy?*
- ❖ *How to take the remedies*
- ❖ *What potency to use*
- ❖ *"Side effects"*
- ❖ *How do we know that it works?*
- ❖ *Homeopathy's best-kept secrets*

*W*hat is homeopathy?

Homeopathy is a scientific method of medicine developed by the German physician Samuel Hahnemann (1755-1843), based on several eternal laws of nature. The first law, *Like cures Like* or the *Law of Similars,* had been formulated centuries earlier by Hippocrates, the father of medicine. A simple example: you have food poisoning and another poison, Arsenic, will bring a speedy recovery (in highly diluted homeopathic doses, of course!). A homeopathic remedy creates a similar (*not the same*) artificial "disease" picture, not the disease itself, but information about the disease which helps the body to organize its defenses. As the body's vital energy pushes back like a rebound effect against the "shadow disease" created by the remedy, it also pushes the actual disease from the inside to the outside.

A homeopathic remedy is thus an almost infinitesimally small dose of a medication which —if given in a bigger dose to a healthy individual—would provoke symptoms similar to those presented by the patient. Western medical doctors often practice "unconscious" homeopathy when they give vaccinations and allergy shots. In general, Western medical treatment is successful when it follows this important *Law of Similars.* Unfortunately, Western science has not made the next important step: applying all the other laws of homeopathy. What are they?

All the remedies used have been "proved" on healthy people: a group of 50 to 100 people take a mild dose of the remedy daily for six weeks and record all their reactions, whether physical, mental or emotional. Clinical experience has shown that the remedy will then be effective in curing these same symptoms in patient. This is the only scientific way of knowing the action of a medication (rather than the conventional method of testing new medications either on sick people whose energy is already depleted, or on animals that cannot report the information needed and, in any case, are different from human beings in their reactions to medications).

In classical homeopathy, remedies are administered one at a time rather than in mixtures. In Western medicine, drugs are usually given in combinations; if the combination works, the doctor does not know which of the drugs to discontinue, so that the patient must suffer the side effects of all of them.

The homeopathic law most puzzling to Western medicine is the smallness of the dose. Most remedies do not possess even one molecule of the original substance. But the remedies maintain and reproduce information about the vibrational pattern of the original substance, just as a CD can reproduce the vibrational pattern of a musical performance, without containing a single molecule of the performer! And the activity of these homeopathic remedies has been demonstrated by rigorous scientific studies. All this shows is that we don't know everything yet about physics and chemistry. I think it is exciting for science that there is still so much to discover.

Furthermore, the quality of a medication has nothing to do with the quantity, which is often dangerous. While there might be a current tendency in Western medicine to prescribe lower doses (again, unconsciously coming closer to homeopathy), the conventional practice is to overprescribe to the limit of toxicity, which leads to antibiotic-resistant bacteria and the resurgence of diseases thought to be conquered long ago.

"Homeopathy? Oh, yes!" a colleague of mine said to me one day. "Those little sugar balls all look the same. How can you heal with them? Placebo, auto-suggestion, maybe charlatanism, that's what homeo-pathy is."

This objection to homeopathy reminds me of the resistance Hahnemann, the founder of homeopathy, encountered from the conventional medical doctors in Paris because they were so threatened by his successes. They asked the minister of medicine, Mr. Guizot, not to allow Hahnemann to practice. This was the wise answer of Mr. Guizot:

Hahnemann is a scientist of great merit. Science is there for everyone. If homeopathy is a system with-

out any ground or value, it will fall by itself. If on the contrary it is progress, it will survive and expand in spite of your efforts. And does not the Medical Academy have the mission of advancing science and encouraging its findings?

A wise answer indeed. And as Hahnemann himself said, the truth always prevails. Homeopathy proved its worth in the great epidemics of contagious diseases in the 19th and early 20th century. Hahnemann saved Napoleon's army from typhoid and conquered the great cholera epidemic of 1831. During the great 1918 flu epidemic, homeopathic hospitals had a mortality rate of only 3%, compared to 45% in the allopathic hospitals.

On the contrary, Western medical drugs are like movie stars: touted briefly as the latest "miracle drug," they are inevitably found to be ineffective or to have unacceptable side effects, and they fade from view after a few years. Homeopathy is here to stay, as long as humankind needs assistance and as long as common sense prevails.

As Dr. Constantine Hering (another giant of homeopathy) said, "Do not accept anything without proving it, *still less* reject anything without trying it." There is nothing better to convince a skeptic regarding the value of homeopathy than the treatment of acute conditions as described in this book.

What would you suggest for someone who wants to get started with homeopathy but feels bewildered by all the different remedies?

Just start with one remedy at a time and get to know all the different things it can be used for. Soon you will feel like the remedies are your friends. Arnica would be my first choice—it's the king of the trauma remedies and king of the sports remedies. Arnica is good for the whole family for bumps, bruises, pulled muscles, and overuse of muscles—like for someone who has a desk job, then gets a two-week vacation and wants to be a hero playing sports with his kids. It's even good for elderly people who get spontaneous bruises, because as we get older the capillaries become fragile and burst easily.

Some lesser known uses of Arnica include overworry; overuse of the voice from speaking all day; and for the flu, especially when there is a bruised feeling. Arnica is for bruises in general, and for illnesses with a bruised feeling, like when you feel as though a tank just ran over you. Everything is sore, and you don't want to be touched.

Arnica is also a great absorber of blood. For example, my patients have had amazing experiences with their kids, who bump their heads and get a big goose-egg on their forehead. This of course means there is a hematoma, a leakage of blood. With Arnica the swelling goes right down and then they don't have to take their kids to the emergency room.

So Arnica is great for the whole family starting from Day One. In fact it's a great remedy *for* Day One! Give Arnica 200C to the mother for bruising from the delivery and give it to the baby for the trauma of coming through the birth canal.

How about another favorite remedy?

Arsenicum would be my second choice, especially for traveling. Never leave home without it! It's the top remedy for traveler's diarrhea and for food poisoning. Some people get diarrhea just from the change of diet when they travel. Arsenicum has rescued many a vacation, especially in the Middle East, China and South America where the water can be contaminated.

Arsenicum is also great for the first stages of a cold or flu, when you are just getting a scratchy throat and your nose is running like a faucet with a clear, watery discharge. Arsenicum will nip it in the bud.

Arsenicum is one of the top remedies for asthma and for shortness of breath in general, especially when you are afraid you are going to die because you can't catch your breath. And it's one of the best remedies for people who wake up after midnight, anxious and restless and unable to get back to sleep. But in both of these cases, people shouldn't diagnose themselves. You really need to see a professional homeopath. For example, in homeopathy we have so many remedies for anxiety. The remedies are very precise, depending on whether the patient has fear of the future, of death, of disease, of failure, of flying, of taking exams, and so on.

What's the best way to take the remedies?

This is one of homeopathy's best-kept secrets: take the remedies in water. When you buy a little tube in the store with 80 pellets, the label says to take 3 pellets 3 to 5 times a day under the tongue. (There is no secret door under the tongue!) But it will work much better and much faster if you take one pellet and dissolve it in 4 ounces of water. (It's best to use purified water—filtered water, spring water or distilled water—but you can use tap water if that's all you have.) *Never touch the pellets with your hands! So don't put them first on your hands and then in your mouth or cup!* You may need to crush the pellet between two clean pieces of paper to dissolve it. Or order the remedy in tiny "poppyseed pellets" from a homeopathic pharmacy; they dissolve right away.

Take one teaspoon or tablespoon as needed—as often as every 15 to 30 minutes in acute cases such as high fevers and accidents. One cup is good for 24 hours. Don't overdo it and take the whole 4 oz. within the first two hours. You would probably have an aggravation (a brief intensification of symptoms, which we try to avoid because it can be uncomfortable). Be sure to slow down to one dose every hour or two as the symptoms improve. And when you are completely well, stop the remedy. Homeopathy is not like Western medicine, which requires you to take antibiotics until they are finished.

If you still need the remedy the next day, make another cup with a new pellet. Putting it in water makes it reach more nerve endings and act more profoundly. As soon as it touches the mucous membranes it starts to work. If someone can't swallow, you can even swab it on their skin—ideally on the lips or another area with many nerve endings close to the surface.

By the way, if someone is hypersensitive (more about that later), they may find taking the remedy in water makes it *too* strong. They may need to take it dry and/or just take a 30c instead of a 200c.

What if you run out of the remedy the same day? Can you make another cup?

You could but you shouldn't need to. As you start to feel better you should slow down and take a teaspoon only maybe every hour or two. Then when the symptoms are gone (or when the person tells you they are feeling fine), *wait* and see if some of the symptoms start appearing again, and only then give another dose of the same remedy. If you don't see any improvement by the time you finish the cup, it probably means you have the wrong remedy. (It could also mean the potency is too low, but this is something you will learn from experience. You may only be able to get a 30C in the health food store, and a strong acute illness in a child, for example, may need 200C.)

So why doesn't the label say to dissolve the remedy in water?

Maybe because they can sell more tubes this way! Or maybe because they just don't know. Hahnemann, the founder of homeopathy, developed this method of taking the remedies in water at the very end of his life, and the manuscript in which he described it was lost for nearly 100 years. Even now it is not well known. The people who manufacture homeopathic remedies may have never read it.

Are there any situations when it's better to take the remedy dry?

Preventively, the remedies should always be taken dry. For most people, the preventive dose is three pellets dry, dissolved in the mouth at once. People who are sensitive to the remedies should only take one pellet.

In acute situations (once you are sick), use a remedy dry only if it's impractical to take it in water. When I play tennis or soccer I keep Arnica and Rhus tox. in my pockets in case I sprain my ankle. I can take some pellets and keep on playing. Then, as soon as I have a chance, I put them in water.

Here's another secret: if you are going to be out all day, driving around in the car, put the remedy in a small water bottle and take it with you. Then each time you take the remedy you can succuss it (give it a hard thwack, a "slam-dunk"). This gradually increases the potency of the remedy and it will work even better this way.

How many pellets, say for a typical 16 oz. bottle of spring water?

Just one. You don't need four just because there is four times as much water. We are dealing with energy, not with molecules. It's a little more dilute this way, but succussing it will keep increasing the potency of the remedy.

Should you reduce the dosage for kids?

Not at all! In fact kids need higher potencies than adults. Never hesitate to give a child a high potency. It's the opposite of Western medicine, where the dosages are based on body weight. In homeopathy the dosage is based on the vital energy of the patient, and kids usually have much stronger vital energy than adults. Look at how fast a child can spike a fever. That shows how strong the vital energy is. To babies, one might only give teaspoons instead of tablespoons, but repetition can be as often as every 10 to 15 minutes. Once there is a positive reaction (a decrease of

11

symptoms, such as a drop in temperature during a fever or a calming effect on the person's mood), you should reduce the frequency of your remedy.

Should I consider changing the remedy if I don't see a change after giving three doses over a time span of two hours?

If you have given enough of the remedy *(see above)* and the symptoms have not changed, it would be prudent to consider a different remedy. At this point it would be wise to consult your homeopathic physician, or check with your regular physician to make sure you have the right diagnosis. If you have a good second choice remedy, you could try it while waiting to reach your homeopath. In fact it is always good to consult with your homeopath if you can, as you will learn from him what to do next in the same situation. In a serious situation, never delay a trip to the emergency room while self-medicating.

Let's say someone looks up in a homeopathy book and figures out that Lachesis is the best remedy for her left-sided headache, but when she goes to the store to buy it, the tube says it's for hot flashes. Why is that?

Each of the major remedies (the polycrests) has many, many different indications or uses. The pharmaceutical company can only fit one or two of them on the label. The good thing is that they have the freedom to do that, unlike vitamin companies, because homeopathic remedies come under a different law and the FDA allows this kind of labeling. So if your homeopathic physician prescribes a remedy, don't be surprised if it says something totally different on that little tube.

Do the remedies have side effects?

No, again because we are talking energy, not molecules. When you use potencies over 12C there is not even one molecule of the original substance left, and then when you put it in water it is even more dilute. You can get what we call a *similar aggravation,* though, if you take too much. An *aggravation* is a temporary intensification of the symptoms. It's unlikely to happen in acute cases, because you are using up the remedy so fast. You would have to really take a lot, maybe 3 or 4 cups of the remedy in a row, to get this kind of reaction.

If you do get an aggravation, just stop taking the remedy and your body will use up the excess. It's like speeding in a car. It's not a bad car, just a bad driver! You need to get used to the car. As you get experience using the remedies, you will get to know how fast you can take repeated doses.

Some people say you have to go through an aggravation to be cured with homeopathy. Would you agree with that?

13

Not at all! Hahnemann developed the water method to save people from the discomfort of aggravations. A similar aggravation always means that you took a little more than you really needed. So you wait until the effect wears off and then take a little less, or take the dose less frequently.

Can you be allergic to the remedies?

No, for the same reason. Sometimes my patients say they can't take Sulphur as a remedy because they are allergic to sulfa drugs. An allergy to sulfa drugs is actually a good indication that the patient *needs* Sulphur! If under the action of a remedy, you get either a discharge or a rash, this proves the remedy is working, as it reflects the healing of the body from the inside to the outside—in other words a cleansing or true healing reaction. Where a rash after administration of a Western medical drug always reflects an allergic reaction, this is *never* the case after the administration of a homeopathic remedy and therefore is *not* a reason to stop the remedy. (However, you can choose to slow down or stop the remedy temporarily if the cleansing reaction is uncomfortable.)

What if someone is allergic to lactose, can they have a reaction to the lactose the pills are made from?

Not usually, but if they are extremely sensitive to lactose they could have a reaction if they take the pills dry. It's another good reason to take the remedies in water as it will decrease that reaction.

You've mentioned taking less of a remedy if you are hypersensitive. How do you know if you are? And how exactly would you change the dosage?

Unfortunately hypersensitivity is a widespread problem in the modern world.You know you are hypersensitive if you suffer from many food allergies; react to perfumes, gasoline exhaust, chemical fumes, and cigarette smoke; and can only take a fraction of the drugs that your doctor prescribes. You are also likely to react to vitamins and to anesthesia.

Often patients complain to me that it took their doctor a lot longer than expected to "wake them up" after an operation. Even worse, many suffer lasting ill effects (such as Chronic Fatigue) from too much anesthesia. A Phosphorus type person, discussed in Part Five, is most likely to be susceptible to anesthesia and its aftereffects. Anyone who is hypersensitive should receive less anesthesia, but unfortunately Western medicine does not recognize this. As a precaution, everyone and especially hypersensitives should take a dose of Phosphorus 200C before dental work or surgery.

If you recognize yourself as one of these sensitive souls, it might be better to take your remedies "dry," in other words, not dissolved in water, and to start with 30C (one pellet as needed) instead of 200C. Also, anywhere you see 3 pellets dry as a dosage, you should automatically take only one. This way you will prevent unwanted aggravations.

Can you develop a tolerance to the remedies the way you can to a drug?

As long as you need the remedy, it will continue to work. If your baby is learning to walk, all the time falling and smacking his head, you can give Arnica every day and it will continue to work. If a remedy stops working, it means you no longer need it. If you keep taking it you could actually get an aggravation of the remedy (which will disappear as soon as you stop the remedy).

Can the remedies be addictive?

There is not one patient in a Betty Ford Center addicted to homeopathic remedies! Whereas there are many treatment centers and detox centers for people addicted to Western drugs. It's scary how easy it is for people to get addicted. All it takes is one hospitalization, where you are given painkillers and sleeping pills without your knowledge or your permission. Before you know it you're addicted. I have seen it many times in my practice.

What do the numbers mean—6C, 30C, 200C?

They represent the successive dilutions the remedies go through. "C" stands for centesimal and it means a dilution of 1 part of the remedy to 99 parts of water/ alcohol at each stage. The remedy is succussed, or shaken, 100 times at each stage so that the vibrational pattern of the remedy is imparted to the liquid. The higher the number, the higher the dilution—which in homeopathy means a more powerful remedy because the vibrational energy is higher.

Usually in health food stores you find 6C, 12C and 30C potencies. What's the difference in how they are used?

I would rather see 30C and 200C in stores, because they are more appropriate for acute (self-limiting) conditions. I encourage my students and patients to get 200C kits once they are familiar with the remedies and how they work. 30C is better when you are first starting out because if you take the wrong remedy in a 200C potency, you could get an uncomfortable aggravation. You definitely should not take a 1M (1,000C) or 10M (10,000C) unless it has been prescribed by a professional homeopath.

6C and 12C are too low to do any good for acute situations, so there is no reason to have them in stores. 6C and 12C are only indicated for chronic diseases, and people should definitely *not* diagnose or treat themselves for chronic diseases. Only a professional homeopathic physician should do that.

Is that because 6C and 12C could be dangerous?

Not at all. But a layperson is not qualified to prescribe for a chronic situation, in which the choice of remedy depends not so much on the physical symptoms as on the mental and emotional onset of the disease. For example, if I have four patients with chronic fatigue, one may be never well since taking birth control pills, another never well since overwork and overworry, another never well since multiple operations, and the fourth never well since heartbreak. Furthermore, they may all have different personalities and underlying constitutions. They may all have the exact same physical symptoms and the same diagnosis in Western medicine, but they will each get a different remedy from me, because homeopathy is so individualized to the patient.

When I have only a 12C potency available, could I just put 3 pellets of 12C in one cup to make it 36C and closer to the 30C you recommend?

No! It does not work that way. Homeopathy does not follow the currently known laws of physics and chemistry. So this kind of arithmetic does not work. Three pellets of a 12C are still a 12C, because it is energy medicine. If you only have a 12C and you want to make it stronger, you have different options:

- Put it in water (4 oz).
- Take a tablespoon or even 2-3 tablespoons at the same time.
- Take it more frequently.
- Put it in a small bottle and succuss it (hit it *hard* on a leather-bound book or the palm of your hand) ten times before you take each dose (1 tablespoon at a time).

What do you mean by acute and chronic illnesses?

An acute condition is something that just happened within the last day or two, within the last several weeks at most, that is self-limiting (it will go away by itself) in most cases. In an acute disease, the vital energy of the patient is usually strong enough to overcome it. If not, it can turn into a chronic condition, one that develops over a long period of time and does not go away by itself. In a chronic condition there can be a steady overall decline in the patient's health unless it is opposed by the right remedy.

Other times there can be acute symptoms of a chronic state of imbalance or disorder in the system, such as PMS. A woman can have acute symptoms each month which can be treated with acute over-the-counter remedies each time—but these acute remedies will do nothing to prevent the recurrence of her symptoms the next month. However, if a professional homeopath treats her overall constitution, her symptoms will not recur because her whole system will return to a balanced state. I have seen this many times in my practice—I do not even address the patient's PMS symptoms directly because they go away automatically with the well-chosen remedy.

A lot of times health food stores have combinations that have 6 or 8 different remedies. Wouldn't that be better than a single remedy, since you would be sure to cover your bases?

Actually, no, because the remedies can cancel each other out. I would rather see people become familiar with the single remedies. For example, I've seen a combination labeled 'Grief' that includes one remedy, Pulsatilla, for people who are very clingy and needy of consolation, and another, Nat. mur., for people who just want to be left alone in their grief. How can one person possibly need both? Furthermore, mixed remedies have not been subjected to a scientific proving. While they sometimes work, Hahnemann condemned this method as unscientific. I do not encourage the use of mixed preparations.

Many homeopaths say you can't use mint, camphor or coffee when you are taking remedies. Would you agree?

Coffee is the only one I put the accent on in my own practice. If someone is drinking more than one cup a day, I get them off the coffee first (with Chamomilla, Nux vomica or Coffea). Decaffeinated coffee and other caffeine-containing foods like chocolate and cola are okay (not in other ways, but in terms of not canceling the remedy!). Mint and camphor are only important when taking the high potencies that are used by the majority of professional homeopaths for chronic illnesses. They won't make much difference in acute situations where you are repeating the doses frequently.

It is better to avoid exposing your remedies to

radiation at airports. Simply pass them to the security people as you would hand over computers, films, etc. It is also wise to avoid exposing your remedies to the sun and other heat sources (for example, in the glove compartment of a car on a hot day).

Don't put a remedy in an empty tube from another remedy, and don't mix it in a cup previously used for a different remedy. The imprint of the previous remedy will still be present. Do not use the same spoon to administer two different remedies; just use a different plastic spoon for each remedy. Take your remedies with a clean mouth, always at least 15 minutes away from food, toothpaste, mouthwash, and strong-flavored drinks. Remember to avoid coffee as it can cancel the remedies.

Do I need to replace my remedies after a certain amount of time or do they stay active for a long time?

Although your remedies may have an expiration date on the label, nothing is further from the truth. Properly stored (that is in a dark, dry, clean and cool place, free from odor and scent, away from sunshine), they stay active *forever*. In fact, remedies from Hahneman's own kit were found to be as active 150 years later as they were in his time.

Should I use external applications of creams to help in the healing process? I'm thinking of the Arnica and Calendula creams which I have seen advertised.

Arnica and Calendula creams can be used safely. But in all honesty, you are going to heal much faster by taking Arnica and Calendula 200C orally, dissolved in water. The same goes for warts—use Thuja internally rather than in cream.

The external application of creams from the drugstore is dangerous because it inevitably suppresses your symptoms, driving the condition deeper inwards with serious chronic disease as a possible consequence. The most common example is the suppression of eczema by cortisone, causing the disorder to go deeper and develop into asthma. Western medicine recognizes a connection between eczema and asthma—but does not understand that the cortisone actually causes it!

For the same reason, one should never use drugs, powders, suppositories or creams to suppress perspiration or discharges, and one should never have warts removed by surgery, cauterization, etc. Treat these conditions homeopathically instead. Otherwise you are blocking the body's natural outlet for a disorder that is deep inside. When a surface outlet is blocked, the body has to discharge it deeper inside, which can lead to a more serious chronic disease.

Some homeopaths tell their patients not to do acupuncture or polarity or take vitamins while on a remedy. Why is that?

I tell my patients to do anything they can to support their vital energy while they are healing. Any healing modality such as acupuncture that follows the same natural laws as homeopathy can only help the healing process. The only thing is, patients shouldn't start doing these things the same week that they start the remedy. This can muddy the picture. Then if they have a reaction (positive or negative), it's not clear what they are reacting to, the acupuncture treatment or the remedy.

Other healing modalities supporting the vital energy include meditation, Tai Chi, QiGong, yoga, chiropractic adjustments, sensible diets and biofeedback. One word of caution about vitamins: they may mask your true energy level and symptoms by artificially enhancing your energy level. Vitamins directed at boosting energy, such as adrenal cortex preparations, should be avoided.

Must I stop my prescription drugs for a chronic disease if I am using homeopathy for an acute illness, or will the remedies still work?

You should never stop your prescription drugs unless advised by your medical doctor. Remedies will still work even when prescription drugs are taken and will *not* interfere with the action of those drugs.

Unfortunately most homeopaths tell their patients they must discontinue their prescription drugs before beginning homeopathic treatment. In my experience with thousands of patients, not only is this unnecessary, it is actually dangerous, because the prescription drug is withdrawn before the remedy can begin to work, leaving the patient vulnerable. It also makes the job of the homeopath more difficult, because the withdrawal symptoms from the drug muddy the picture and make it more difficult to discern whether the remedy is working.

I've heard that remedies are prescribed based on the patient's symptoms. So does that mean the remedies can't be used preventively?

No, in fact here's another little-known tip. They can be used ahead of time if you expect to need them, but in this case take 3 pellets dry in the mouth instead of in water. For example, Arnica should be taken before and after strenuous sports by someone who is not in shape, or by weight lifters, football players, soccer players and others who are likely to get pulled muscles or bruises.

And if one person in the family comes down with a flu or cold, everyone else in the family can take the same remedy. When you mix up the remedy cup for the sick person, give a teaspoon to everyone else in the house every day. If you know there is a flu coming to your area, you can start taking Arsenicum or Oscillococcinum (the two top preventive flu remedies) before it even hits. Take 200C doses, 3 pellets dry once a week during an epidemic, or even once a day if you are exposed to the flu on a daily basis (for example if you work with people who have the flu).

Does homeopathy work on animals too?

Absolutely! It should make a believer out of any skeptic who claims that it is just a placebo effect. Dogs, cats, horses, birds ... they don't know what you give them (nor do one-day-old infants, yet it works on babies too!). Acute remedies work fabulously for animals, and I hope you can find a homeopathic vet to help you with some of your pets' more serious, chronic problems. But homeopathy will treat the acute events described very effectively, to the delight and comfort of your beloved animals.

Should we buy these remedies in single tubes as we need them, or would you advise us to buy a homeopathic kit with 25 to 50 remedies?

When you are just sticking your toes in the water, so to speak, get 30C potencies as you need them at the health food store. Then when you have experience with the remedies and feel ready to work with 200Cs, you should definitely get a 200C emergency kit. Then when you phone your doctor you have the remedies ready, even late at night or after midnight. And pricewise a kit is a bargain since each remedy costs about $5, while the whole kit with 50 remedies costs less than $100! And you will never have to buy another kit for the rest of your life. The cost of an average homeopathic treatment is only *one cent* per day! The whole family will benefit from it. It certainly would be a nice present to give a kit along with this book to any friend. This is what I would recommend for a homeopathic 200C emergency kit.

Aconitum	*Ferrum phosphoricum*
Allium cepa	*Gelsemium*
Antimonium tartaricum	*Hamamelis*
Apis	*Hepar sulphur*
Argentum nitricum	*Hydrastis*
Arnica montana	*Ignatia*
Arsenicum album	*Ipecac*
Belladonna	*Kali bichromicum*
Bryonia	*Lycopodium*
Calendula	*Mercurius vivus*
Cantharis	*(Mercurius solubilis)*
Capsicum	*Nux vomica*
Carbo vegetalis	*Phosphorus*
Causticum	*Pulsatilla*
Chamomilla	*Rhus toxicodendron*
China	*Ruta graveolens*
Cina	*Sanguinaria*
Cocculus	*Silicea*
Colocynthis	*Spigelia*
Cuprum metallicum	*Spongia*
Drosera	*Sulphur*
Euphrasia	*Veratrum album*

Is there any proof that homeopathy works?

First of all, just like acupuncture, it has stood the test of time. If something does not work, it will not last. Western medicine should abandon its attacks on alternative medicines: if they have no merit, they will crumble by themselves. The great effectiveness of homeopathy has been documented for the last two hundred years. It has been triumphant in both acute and chronic illnesses. As Hahnemann himself so well demonstrated, it can even conquer the most devastating epidemics: cholera, scarlat fever, typhoid fever, etc.

But Western medicine demands "double-blind" studies in which neither the patient nor doctor knows whether the patient receives the medicine or a placebo (an inert look-alike).

First, such studies *have* been performed, and have proved the effectiveness of homeopathic remedies in conditions such as hay fever, children's diarrheas and head traumas. Scientists who claim that homeopathy is "unproven" are simply ignorant of these studies, which unfortunately are mostly published abroad and are not yet included in any American medical school curriculum.

Furthermore, the double-blind studies are fundamentally limited or erroneous. First of all, they are funded by drug companies, which are not willing to pay millions of dollars to show that inexpensive, non-patentable homeopathic remedies work better than their expensive drugs. After all, pharmaceutical companies are in the business of making money.

Then the basic premise of a double-blind study goes against the basic laws of homeopathy. In a double-blind study all the patients receive the same drug, but one of the strengths of homeopathy is that we individualize the remedy to the patient. Western medicine categorizes patients by the disease name. In homeopathy we do not prescribe for a disease name but for the person with the disease.

Another stumbling block is that double-blind studies are conducted on sick people whose vital energy is already weakened. In the past thousands of people have died from these experiments. Or we test these drugs on animals. How do we know that humans will react in the same fashion? Even worse, animals cannot communicate the mental and emotional changes they feel under the effects of drugs. But these are always the first signs of illness, showing up *before* physical changes detected by lab tests. In other words, Western medicine waits until the *last* stage of the disease, the *pathological* changes, to draw conclusions.

Far *more scientific* is the method of "proving" homeopathic remedies. Each remedy was given in a 30C potency for six weeks to a *healthy* cross-section of adults (about 50 people). Their symptoms (mental, emotional and physical) were noted in the provers' own words. (To show the courage of homeopathic physicians, they conducted the first provings on themselves, quite the contrary of Western medicine in which painful experimental procedures are sometimes "practiced" on dying patients.) The information gathered from the provings was organized into repertories such as the mini-version in this manual. The proof of the method is that if the provers showed a symptom from a remedy, that same remedy will relieve that symptom in an ill person.

So let us not force ill-conceived tests on the truly scientific method of homeopathy, which follows the infallible healing Laws of Nature.

You are both a homeopath and an acupuncturist. What do you see as the connection between these two healing modalities?

They both work with the healing energy or vital *Qi*, and they both follow the same natural laws of healing. For example, we know the patient is healing if the disease goes from the inside to the outside, for example a chronic disease will turn into a skin rash or discharge. Also both disciplines emphasize the mental and emotional origins of disease (unless of course there is a direct physical trauma like a cut, blow or burn). In both, each organ has certain emotions associated with it, such as the liver with anger. Each of the main homeopathic remedies has a place on the Star of the Five Elements in Traditional Chinese Medicine. Homeopathy is so similar to acupuncture that we believe Hahnemann must have read the acupuncture texts that were available to him in translation.

29

Does someone have to be a medical doctor to practice homeopathy?

In terms of licensing, it varies from state to state. In terms of knowledge, many of the greatest homeopaths have been lay people.

Any parting thoughts?

Never force your beliefs upon other people. You can suggest a homeopathic remedy to someone for an acute case, but don't force it upon them. If they want it, they can experience the magic of homeopathy with you. There is a Chinese saying, "Don't teach until you are asked." Respect for people is an expression of love.

For more questions and answers on homeopathy, read my book **Human Condition: Critical,** *available at your health food store or from Full of Life Publishing (see ordering information at the back of the book).*

PART TWO

How to Use the Repertory

- ❖ *Taking the case*
- ❖ *Selecting the remedy*
- ❖ *Practical examples*

THREE THINGS ARE EQUALLY IMPORTANT in homeopathy—taking the case (getting information from the patient), selecting the remedy, and administering the remedy. These three steps are very closely intermingled. How to administer remedies in acute cases has been covered in Part One. Now we will address the other two components: taking the case and selecting the remedy.

Taking the case

There is a huge difference between taking a chronic case and an acute case. As we emphasized before, the layperson should *never* attempt to do a chronic case; leave that instead to your professional homeopath. But there are numerous acute, self-limiting events in your daily life which you can safely and successfully treat with homeopathy.

In Western medicine we tend to lump diseases together into large categories with a single disease name, whereas in homeopathy the remedies are highly individualized both to the patient and to the exact nature of the disease. In Western medicine, if you have a cough, the cough syrup you choose has a lot more to do with what was most marketed (on TV or at your doctor's office) and which one has the best taste. When I ask my patients, "What kind of cough do you have?" I am inevitably met with a blank stare.

"What do you mean, doctor, a cough is a cough, isn't it? If you want to know, it's a hell of a cough!" As you will see from this mini-version of the repertory, "a hell of a cough" is a symptom which won't help you select the right remedy because you won't find it! One of the strengths of homeopathy is that it individualizes—in other words, it differentiates among all kinds of coughs, making your kind of cough unique, responding only to the right remedy.

In the case of an acute illness we just need **three important symptoms** to select our remedy (we call it the "three-legged stool"). Often we ask questions like:

- *Where?* Where is the complaint located?
- *Sensation?* What is the sensation, how does it feel? "As if...."; is it sharp, bruised, blunt, etc.
- *When?* The time when the symptom starts, recurs or improves is important.
- *What* affects the complaints for *better or worse?* (For example, a headache may be worse with the slightest movement, bright light, or a draft; it may feel better from an ice pack or firm pressure.)
- *Why?* What caused the disease? Was it an emotional event like hearing bad news or a physical trauma (overlifting, fall, etc.)?
- What are symptoms *accompanying* this main symptom? e.g. headaches with flickering lights; diarrhea with vomiting; dizziness with nausea.

33

Selecting the remedy

The different symptoms you might have are all arranged in what we call "rubrics." In a homeopathic repertory, you can look up a rubric and find a group of remedies which have been shown to relieve this symptom. Sometimes, under the chief rubric, there is what we call a "subrubric." This is used to narrow down the choice of our remedy. It is a symptom listed below the main symptom as a modifier of that main rubric.

For instance, let's say our complaint is an animal bite. We will find "Bite," the chief rubric, but then we will also have subrubrics, like "cats," "dogs," and "mosquitoes" (i.e., the bites of these different species). In other words, they make our remedy choice more precise. The rubrics are listed in alphabetical order. In a full-length repertory you will find many more remedies for each rubric. However, I have limited the amount of entries in each rubric to the most common remedies for that condition, to simplify the choices for the lay prescriber.

The different remedies are written in either **bold type** (the most important remedies, which should be your first choice), *italics* (second most important) or regular print (least important). For example, **Bryonia** is listed in bold type under "Headaches," because it is a remedy very frequently and successfully employed for headaches (especially those worse with the slightest movement, as the subrubric indicates).

Once you have selected your remedy, you need to read about it in Part Four, *A Guide to the Remedies*. This is especially important if you are trying to decide between two or three remedies. See *Practical Examples* below.

The Repertory part is divided into different sections arranged in the following order:

- **MENTAL** covers all emotional events, temperaments, emotional states such as fears, anxieties, anger, etc.

- **EMERGENCY** covers emergencies as well as typical home uses like cuts, bruises, burns, sprains, strains, indigestion, etc.

- **COUGHS, COLDS and FLUS** has several different headings: *Cough, Expectoration* (indicating the kind of mucus brought up), *Colds* (with the different stages of a cold, starting in the nose and progressing deeper to the throat or chest), *Throat,* and *Flu* with the common remedies for treating and preventing the flu. (The dosage for prevention: use a 200C of the remedy, 3 pellets dry, once a week if the flu is in your general vicinity; daily if you have limited exposure, e.g. from someone at work; and if someone in your family or living situation is ill, take a teaspoon of their remedy daily from their dosage cup.)

- **WOMEN'S HEALTH** includes remedies for menses, pregnancy, delivery, and other health concerns for women.

Practical examples of using the repertory

1. You just injured your back. In the "Emergency" section, you look for "Back" in alphabetical order, and you find:

BACK injuries: **Arn., Bry., Hyper.,Rhus-t.,** *Ruta*
    dislocations: **Arn., Bry., Rhus-t.**
    disks, slipped, herniated: **Bry., Hyper.**
    lifting, from: **Arn., Bry., Hyper., Rhus-t.**
    straining (lumbago): **Rhus-t.,** *Ruta*

First you will see the main rubric with the remedies Arnica, Bryonia, Hypericum, Rhus tox. and Ruta. (The key to the abbreviations is in the beginning of Part Three, *The Repertory.*) Which one to choose? You might either read up on each remedy in the *Guide to the Remedies.* Or even better, you can look in the subrubrics where the injury is explained more in depth: from dislocations, from overlifting, from straining ... or is it a slipped disc, which you would know by the numbness and tingling in the leg? As you can see, each of these subrubrics have their own remedies. You can narrow down your choices and then read about them in the *Guide to the Remedies.*

2. You just heard over the phone that your best friend died in an accident. You are shocked and dazed. We call this "hearing bad news." Look up this rubric under the "Mental" section and you will find:

BAD NEWS, hearing: **Gels.**, *Ign.*

When you look up the two main remedies, Gelsemium and Ignatia, in the *Guide to the Remedies*, you will see that the person who needs Gelsemium reacts with trembling, drowsiness, dizziness and feels paralyzed. Someone who needs Ignatia, on the other hand, reacts with "sitting, sighing, and sobbing"; in other words she becomes over-emotional, lamenting what has happened. It will be easy to make your choice based on your emotional reaction and how you express it.

3. You just came down with a cold, accompanied by a cough which is worse when you are exposed to cold air. Your section, obviously, is "Cough." The main rubric is "AIR, < cold," while you have a subrubric, "< when going from warm to cold air." (The abbreviation < means "feels worse from" or "the condition is made worse by.")

AIR:
> < cold: **Hep., Phos., Rumex**
> < dry, cold: **Acon., Hep.**
> < going from warm to cold: *Phos.,* **Rumex**

Under the subrubric you will find two remedies, Phosphorus and Rumex. You could read about these remedies in your *Guide to the Remedies* to make your choice. You could also search further under "Cough" for other rubrics/subrubrics which contain Phosphorus or Rumex to help you narrow down your choice. For example, you cough so hard you can't even talk. You find the rubric, "Talking, inability to speak, with," which contains Rumex but not Phosphorus, and that clinches your choice.

For coughs in general, you might go over all the different rubrics of cough to determine which ones apply to you. The remedy which appears in the most rubrics pertaining to "your kind of a cough" is the one which will help the most. For example, you have a barking, choking cough which gets worse when you breathe in cold air. It also sounds croupy and dry, especially at night. Hepar sulph. will be your first choice when you consider all the above rubrics (barking, choking, < in cold air, croupy, dry, at night). Here are your rubrics, and notice that Hepar sulph. (Hep.) is the only remedy that appears in all of them:

AIR:
> < cold: **Hep., Phos., Rumex**
> < dry, cold: **Acon., Hep.**

BARKING (like a seal): **Acon., Bell., Dros., Hep., Spong.**

CHOKING: Alum., Coc-c., Hep., **Ip.,** *Kali-bi., Lach.*

CROUPY: Acon., Hep., Kali-bi., Phos., *Rumex,* **Samb., Spong.**

DRY: Acon., Alum., Ars., Bell., Bry., Hep., Nux-v., Phos., Puls., Rumex, Spong.

night: **Ars., Bell., Dros., Hep., Phos., Puls., Spong., Sulph.**

This may seem a little tricky at first with all the abbreviations. But each time you use a homeopathic remedy and you see how it works, you will make a new friend, and soon all these unfamiliar abbreviations will seem like old friends.

How to communicate your case to your physician by telephone, letter, fax, or e-mail:

Even for acute care, you will learn quite a bit from your homeopathic physician, assuming you are giving him the correct information. This is like learning a new language which requires you, the patient, to pay more attention to your complaints and to give more details than you would to your Western doctor.

First you need to describe your symptoms in your own words, as if you were not familiar with these instructions. Describe your condition: its onset, progress and possible cause. Try to describe your appearance, or have a family member describe you. How is your complexion, your color? Try to describe your *mental/emotional* state, or have a family member describe you: suffering patiently; clingy, crying, looking for consolation; or wanting to be left alone; mild and yielding; or in despair, anxious, irritable, or even delirious with fever (someone else will need to report this!).

39

Next you need to describe your symptoms accurately and completely, beginning with the part and side of the body and how large a space is affected. Try to say in your own words what "kind of" pain or sensation you have: tickling, piercing, dull, sore, twitching, sharp, tearing, throbbing, pulsating, etc. This is very important for your homeopath.

Are the symptoms continuous or do they come and go? Did they start suddenly or come on gradually? Do they recur at any given time of day or night? Are the complaints affected by rest, movement, exercise, bending over, lying down, sitting, walking, noise, light, or touch? And if by touch, is it light or firm pressure? Is the weather playing a role: cold air, wind, humidity? Are your hearing and vision affected? Does a symptom in one part of the body alternate with another one somewhere else?

Try to be as specific as you can about your symptoms. Is there dryness of the mouth or increased salivation? Thirst with fever, or the more uncommmon lack of thirst? Is the breathing short or oppressed, rattling or asthmatic? Is there a cough? Is it hard and dry or is there expectoration of mucus? If so, what color and consistency (thin, ropy, thick, stringy, etc.)? Is it easy to bring up or difficult? How does the mucus taste: salt, sweet, bitter?

Is there itching of the skin? If so, is it relieved by scratching, or do you scratch until it bleeds? Is the itching worse after a hot shower, in bed or when exposed to cold air when undressing?

Is your sleep disturbed, and if so how? When do you wake up and why? Do you have anxious dreams? In what position do you sleep?

This is the type of information your homeopath needs to individualize the remedy to you, the patient. Once you see how perfectly the remedies are fit to the person in homeopathy, Western medicine will seem limited in its attempt to group people into diagnosis categories and then treat them all with the same protocol.

Overwhelming? Maybe just a little at first, but soon you will find out how easy it is. Your homeopath can help you, but your own careful reading and practice with the Repertory will is the best way to experience the "magic of the minimum dose"! Homeopathy will not disappoint you.

One warning: getting to know homeopathy is infectious; it will change your life!

PART THREE

The Repertory

Note: *All the conditions described are for acute, limited care. This repertory should not be used for chronic conditions (see Part One). I also encourage you to consult your physician even for apparently harmless acute cases: cuts, traumas, foreign objects in the eye, burns, etc. Recurring headaches, for example, could be caused by a brain tumor. But by immediately applying the remedies for first aid that are explained in this book, valuable time and healing energy will be gained.*

Remedies and Their Abbreviations

Acon.	Aconitum napellus
Agar.	Agaricus muscarius
All-c.	Allium cepa
Alum.	Aluminum
Ambr.	Ambrosia
Anac.	Anacardium orientale
Ant-c.	Antimonium crudum
Ant-t.	Antimonium tartaricum
Apis	Apis mellifica
Arg-n.	Argentum nitricum
Arn.	Arnica montana
Ars.	Arsenicum album
Arum-t.	Arum triphyllum
Aur.	Aurum metallicum
Bapt.	Baptisia tinctoria
Bell.	Belladonna
Bell-p.	Bellis perennis
Berb.	Berberis vulgaris
Bry.	Bryonia alba
Cact.	Cactus grandiflorus
Cadm.	Cadmium sulphuratum
Calc.	Calcarea carbonica
Calc-p.	Calcarea phosphorica
Calen.	Calendula officinalis
Canth.	Cantharis
Caps.	Capsicum
Carb-ac.	Carbolic acid
Carbo-v.	Carbo vegetalis

Caul.	Caulophyllum
Caust.	Causticum
Cham.	Chamomilla
Chin.	China officinalis
Chin-a.	Chininum arsenicosum
Cimic.	Cimicifuga racemosa
Cina	Cina
Coca	Coca
Cocc.	Cocculus indicus
Coc-c.	Coccus cacti
Coff.	Coffea tosta
Colch.	Colchicum autumnale
Coloc.	Colocynthis
Cupr.	Cuprum metallicum
Dros.	Drosera rotundifolia
Dulc.	Dulcamara
Equis.	Equisetum hiemale
Eup-per.	Eupatorium perfoliatum
Euphr.	Euphrasia
Ferr-p.	Ferrum phosphoricum
Gels.	Gelsemium sempervirens
Glon.	Glonoin
Hep.	Hepar sulphuris
Hydr.	Hydrastis canadensis
Hyper.	Hypericum perforatum
Ign.	Ignatia amara
Ip.	Ipecacuanha
Jab.	Jaborandi
Kali-bi.	Kali bichromicum

Kali-p.	Kali phosphoricum
Kreos.	Kreosotum
Lac-c.	Lac caninum
Lac-d.	Lac defloratum
Lach.	Lachesis
Led.	Ledum palustre
Lyc.	Lycopodium clavatum
Mag-p.	Magnesia phosphorica
Merc.	Mercurius vivus (solubilis)
Mez.	Mezereum
Mur-ac.	Muriaticum acidum
Nat-m.	Natrum muriaticum
Nat-s.	Natrum sulphuricum
Nit-ac.	Nitric acidum
Nux-v.	Nux vomica
Petr.	Petroleum
Ph-ac.	Phosphoricum acidum
Phos.	Phosphorus
Phyt.	Phytolacca decandra
Podo.	Podophyllum
Puls.	Pulsatilla
Ran-b.	Ranunculus bulbosus
Rhus-t.	Rhus toxicodendron
Rumex	Rumex crispus
Ruta	Ruta graveolens
Sabad.	Sabadilla
Samb.	Sambucus nigra
Sang.	Sanguinaria canadensis
Sars.	Sarsaparilla

Sep.	Sepia
Sil.	Silicea
Sol.	Solanum nigrum
Spig.	Spigelia marilandica
Spong.	Spongia tosta
Stann.	Stannum metallicum
Staph.	Staphysagria
Sul-ac.	Sulphuricum acidum
Sulph.	Sulphur
Symph.	Symphytum officinale
Tab.	Tabacum
Tarent-c.	Tarentula cubensis
Urt-u.	Urtica urens
Verat.	Veratrum album
Zinc.	Zincum metallicum

Common Abbreviations

agg.: aggravate, feel worse from, symptoms intensify from

amel.: ameliorate, feel better from, symptoms are relieved by

< worse from (aggravated by)

> better from (ameliorated by)

< > opposite of *(used when one remedy has the opposite effect or opposite action from another; for example, Rhus tox. is a remedy commonly used when rheumatic complaints are worse from dampness; Causticum has the opposite quality of rheumatic complaints that get better in damp weather.)*

ABANDONED, feeling: Aur., Ign., Puls.

**ANGER: Cham., Merc., Nux-v., Sep., Sil.,
Sulph.**

    answer, when forced to: **Nux-v.**

    blamed, when being: Ign.

    contradiction, from: **Aur., Ign., Lyc., Sep.**

    menses, before: *Sep.*

    harassed, from being: **Coloc., Ign.,** *Lyc.,*
       Nux-v., Staph.

    work, about: **Nux-v.**

**ANXIETY: Arg-n., Ars., Aur., Chin., Lyc.,
Nit-ac., Phos., Puls., Sulph.**

    anticipation, from: **Arg-n.,** Gels.

    breathing, from difficult: **Ars., Spong.**

    business, about: **Nux-v.**

    dreams, on waking from frightful: **Acon.,** *Ars.*

    money, matters about: *Ars., Aur.*

    pains, from: *Acon.,* **Ars.,** *Coloc.*

    riding downhill: **Bor.**

    thunderstorm, during: **Phos.**

BAD NEWS, hearing: Gels., *Ign.*

BUSINESS, averse to: *Puls.,* **Sep.,** *Sulph.*

CAPRICIOUS: Cham., Cina, *Puls.,* **Staph.**

CARRIED, desires to be: Cham., *Cina, Lyc.*

EXCITEMENT (too much joy): **Coffea**

EXHAUSTION from mental work: Kali-p.

FEAR: Acon., Arg-n., Gels., Phos.

agoraphobia: *Acon., Arg-n., Ign.*

AIDS or cancer, of: **Ars., Nit-ac.**

airplanes, flying in: **Arg-n.,** *Gels.*

dentist, of: **Gels.**

dogs, of: **Bell., Chin.**

earthquake, after, trembling from: **Gels.**

happen, something will: *Ars.,* **Caust., Phos.,**
    Staph.

fright, sudden: **Acon., Gels., Ign.**

public speaking, of: **Arg-n., Gels., Lyc.**

suffering, of (physical pain): **Aur.**

GRIEF: Aur., Caust., Ign., *Ph-ac.,* **Puls.,** *Staph.*

silent (cannot cry): **Ign.,** *Puls.*

HOMESICKNESS: Caps., Ph-ac.

HUMILIATION (being put down, abuse): *Caust.,*
Coloc., **Staph.**

INSOMNIA

children, in: **Carc., Coff.**

cramps in calves, from : *Cupr., Mag-p.*

excitement, from: **Coff.**

fright, from: **Acon.**

grief, from: **Ign.**

humiliation, from: *Coloc.*

nursing a loved one, from: *Caust.,* **Cocc.,** *Ph-ac.*

overeating, from: **Chin., Nux-v.**

overwork, mental, from: **Nux-v.**

pains, from: **Cham.**

restless feet, from : **Zinc.**

strong coffee, from: **Coff., Nux-v.**

INSOMNIA, *continued:*
> thoughts, activity of: **Coff.**
> toothache or dentition, from: **Cham., Kreos.**
> waking at 3 a.m.: **Nux-v.**
> wine, after drinking too much: **Nux-v.**, *Zinc.*

LOVE, disappointments in: *Aur.,* **Ign., Ph-ac.,** *Staph.*
> silent grief (cannot cry): **Ign., Ph-ac.**

MENTAL EXHAUSTION: Aur., Kali-p., Nux-v., Ph-ac., Phos., Sep., Sulph.
> reading, from: *Sil.*
> talking, from: *Calc-p.*
> writing, after: *Sil.*
> overstudy, from: **Kali-p.**

SADNESS: Ars., Aur., Caust., Ign., Puls., Sep.
> bad news, after: *Ign., Puls.*
> business, when thinking of: *Puls.*
> menses, before: **Puls.,** *Sep.*
> during: *Puls., Sep.*

SENSITIVE, oversensitive:
> noise, to: **Coff., Nux-v., Sil.**
> rudeness, to: **Staph.**

WEEPING: Apis, Caust., Ign., *Ph-ac.,* **Puls., Sep.**
> carried, is quiet when: **Cham.**
> for no reason: **Puls.,** *Sep.*
> joy, from: *Coff.*
> menses, before: *Phos., Puls.*
> during: *Ign., Puls., Sep.*
> pains, with bad: *Coff.*

Emergency

ABSCESS: Hep., Sil.
> foreign bodies, promotes elimination of: **Sil.**

ALLERGIC, reactions:
> hives: **Apis, Ars., Urt-u.**
> runny nose (rhinitis): **All-c., Euphr., Nux-v.**

ALTITUDE sickness: **Carb-v., Coca,** *Sil.*

AMPUTATION, pain after: *All-c.,* **Coff., Hyper.**

BACK injuries: **Arn., Bry., Hyper., Rhus-t., Ruta**
> dislocations: **Arn., Bry., Rhus-t.**
> disks, slipped or herniated: **Bry., Hyper.**
> lifting, from: **Arn., Bry., Hyper., Rhus-t.**
> straining (lumbago): **Rhus-t.,** *Ruta*

BEDWETTING: Equis., Kreos., Puls.

BITES, animals and insects, from:
> bees: **Apis, Carb-ac.**
> cats, of: **Hyper., Led.**
> dogs, of: **Bell.,** *Calen., Hyper., Led.*
> fleas: **Led.**
> mosquitoes: **Led.,** *Staph.*
> burn, itch intensely: *Calad.*
> scorpions: **Hyper., Led.**
> spiders: **Led.**
> wasps: **Apis**

BLADDER, burning sensation:
> cystitis: **Canth.**
> catheter, after: **Staph.**

BLEEDING: Ferr-p., Ip., Phos.
> gums, after dental intervention: **Phos.**

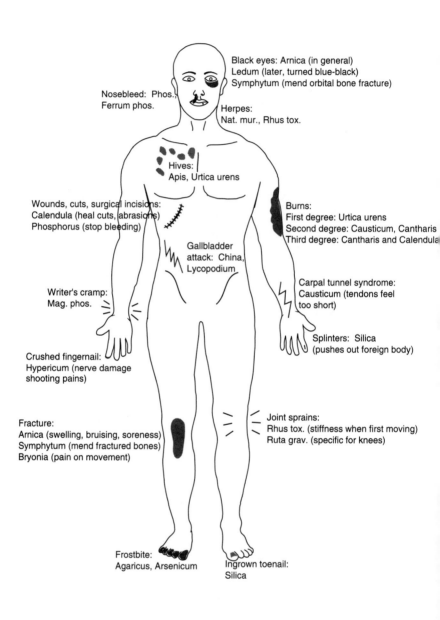

Black eyes: Arnica (in general)
Ledum (later, turned blue-black)
Symphytum (mend orbital bone fracture)

Nosebleed: Phos.
Ferrum phos.

Herpes:
Nat. mur., Rhus tox.

Hives:
Apis, Urtica urens

Wounds, cuts, surgical incisions:
Calendula (heal cuts, abrasions)
Phosphorus (stop bleeding)

Burns:
First degree: Urtica urens
Second degree: Causticum, Cantharis
Third degree: Cantharis and Calendula

Gallbladder
attack: China,
Lycopodium

Writer's cramp:
Mag. phos.

Carpal tunnel syndrome:
Causticum (tendons feel
too short)

Crushed fingernail:
Hypericum (nerve damage
shooting pains)

Splinters: Silica
(pushes out foreign body)

Fracture:
Arnica (swelling, bruising, soreness)
Symphytum (mend fractured bones)
Bryonia (pain on movement)

Joint sprains:
Rhus tox. (stiffness when first moving)
Ruta grav. (specific for knees)

Frostbite:
Agaricus, Arsenicum

Ingrown toenail:
Silica

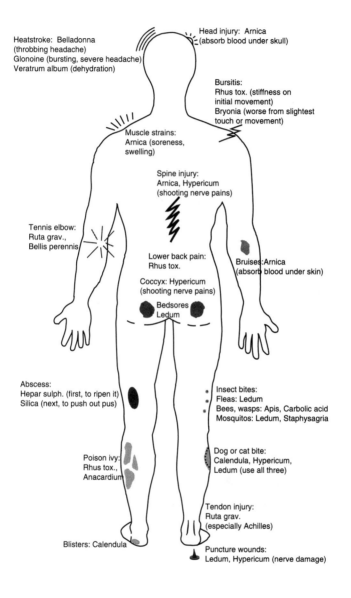

Heatstroke: Belladonna
(throbbing headache)
Glonoine (bursting, severe headache)
Veratrum album (dehydration)

Head injury: Arnica
(absorb blood under skull)

Bursitis:
Rhus tox. (stiffness on
initial movement)
Bryonia (worse from slightest
touch or movement)

Muscle strains:
Arnica (soreness,
swelling)

Spine injury:
Arnica, Hypericum
(shooting nerve pains)

Tennis elbow:
Ruta grav.,
Bellis perennis

Lower back pain:
Rhus tox.

Coccyx: Hypericum
(shooting nerve pains)

Bruises: Arnica
(absorb blood under skin)

Bedsores
Ledum

Abscess:
Hepar sulph. (first, to ripen it)
Silica (next, to push out pus)

Insect bites:
Fleas: Ledum
Bees, wasps: Apis, Carbolic acid
Mosquitos: Ledum, Staphysagria

Poison ivy:
Rhus tox.,
Anacardium

Dog or cat bite:
Calendula, Hypericum,
Ledum (use all three)

Tendon injury:
Ruta grav.
(especially Achilles)

Blisters: Calendula

Puncture wounds:
Ledum, Hypericum (nerve damage)

BLEEDING *continued*:

 nose, from: *Arn., Ferr-p., Mill.,* **Phos.**

 surgery, after: *Calen.*

 trauma, after: **Arn.**

BLISTERS: Calen.

 herpes-like: **Rhus-t.**

BOILS: Sil., Tarent-c.

BREAST, injury from blow to: *Arn.,* **Bell-p., Con.**

BRUISES: Arn., Led., Phos., Ruta

 blunt instrument, from: **Arn**

 contusion: **Arn., Led.**

 crushing tips of fingers: **Hyper.**

 eye, black: **Led., Symph.**

BURNS: Ars., *Calen.,* **Canth.,** *Caust.,* **Sol., Urt-u.**

 1st degree: **Urt-u.**

 2nd degree: **Canth., Caust.**

 3rd degree: **Calen., Canth.** *(hospitalization required!)*

 sun, from: **Canth., Sol.**

CANKER SORES (aphthae): **Bor., Merc., Nux-v.**

CHILDREN'S DISEASES:

 chicken pox: **Ant-t., Puls.**

 impetigo: **Ant-c.**

 measles: **Puls.**

 mumps: *Jab.,* **Puls.**

 rubella (German measles): **Puls.**

COFFEE

withdrawal headaches: **Cham.**, *Coff.*, *Nux-v.*

insomnia, from: **Coff.**, **Nux-v.**

cramps, in stomach, from: **Nux-v.**

COLIC, in babies: **Arg-n, Coloc., Lyc.**

CONSTIPATION: **Alum., Bry., Lyc., Nux-v., Sil., Sulph.**

children: **Nux-v.**

desire, with constant: **Nux-v.**

drugs, after abuse of: **Nux-v.**

sedentary habits, from: *Lyc.,* **Nux-v.**

travel, while on: *Lyc., Nux-v.*

CUTS: **Calen.**, *Hyper.,* **Staph.**

sharp instruments, glass: **Calen.**

DIARRHEA:

alcoholic drinks, from: **Nux-v.**

anxiety, anticipation, from: **Arg-n.**

bad news, after hearing: *Gels.*

dentition, during: **Cham.**

fright, from: **Gels.**

fruit, from: **Ars., Chin.,Verat.**

ice cream, from: **Ars.**, *Puls.*

periodically, on alternate days: **Chin.**

sugar, from: **Arg-n**.

waking, upon: *Nat-s.,* **Sulph.**

wet, after getting: **Rhus-t.**

EAR INFECTIONS

right side: **Bell., Cham., Puls.**

left side: **Graph., Puls.**

with greenish, yellow thick discharge: **Merc.**

ELBOW, injury (tendinitis): **Bell-p., Ruta**

ELECTRIC SHOCK: Phos.

EYES, injuries: **Acon., Arn., Calen., Hyper., Symph.**

> black eye: **Arn., Led.**
>
> blow to, with fracture: **Symph.**
>
> foreign object, splinter: **Acon., Hyper., Sil.**

FALLS: Arn., Calen., Hyper., Nat-s., Ruta, *Symph.*

> head, on: **Arn., Nat-s.**

FOOD POISONING: Ars., *Chin.,* **Puls.**

FRACTURES: Arn., Bry., *Calc-p.,* **Symph.**

FROSTBITE: Agar., *Ars., Nux-v., Puls.*

GALLBLADDER, pain: **Chin., Lyc.**

GOUT, acute attack: *Colch.,* **Urt-u.**

HANGOVER after:

> beer: **Nux-v.**
>
> whiskey: **Led.**
>
> wine: **Zinc.**

HEADACHES: Bry., Coff., Gels., Ign., Ip., *Lyc.,* **Nat-s., Nux-v., Sang., Sil.,** *Spig.*

> both eyes, above: **Sil.**
>
> head trauma: **Arn.**
>
> left-sided: **Bry., Spig.**
>
> maldigestion, from: **Lyc.**
>
> menses, before: **Bry.**
>
> overstudy, from: **Calc-p.**
>
> right-sided: **Lyc., Sang.**
>
> sinus headache: **Hydr., Kali-bi., Puls.**
>
> sun, exposure: **Bell., Glon.**

HERPES (cold sores): **Nat-m., Rhus-t.**

Herpes zoster (shingles): **Ran-b., Rhus-t.**

HIVES (urticaria): **Apis, Ars., Urt-u.**

fish, from: **Ars., Urt-u.**

strawberries, from: **Apis**

fruit or ice cream, from: **Ars.**

JET LAG: *Arn.,* **Cocc.,** *Gels.*

KIDNEY STONES: **Berb., Sars., Sul-ac.**

KNEE, injury: **Arn., Bry., Rhus-t., Ruta**

LIGHTNING, struck by: **Phos.**

LOSS OF FLUIDS (diarrhea, blood, etc.): **Chin.,** *Ph-ac.*

MOTION sickness: **Cocc., Nux-v., Petr., Sep., Tab.**

boat, while in: **Petr., Tab.**

car, riding in: **Cocc.**

plane, in: **Cocc.**

MUSCLE cramps: **Colc., Cupr., Mag-p.**

NAILS, injuries:

crushed: **Hyper.**

splinters, from: **Sil., Hyper.**

NAUSEA: *Ars., Cadm.,* **Ip.,** *Nux-v.,* **Tab.**

chemotherapy, after: **Cadm.,** *Ip.*

constant: **Ip.**

overeating, after: **Nux-v.**

vomiting does not relieve: **Ip.**

OVERLIFTING, injury from: *Arn.,* **Rhus-t.**

POISON OAK or IVY: **Anac., Rhus-t.**

PUNCTURE wounds: **Apis, Calen., Hyper., Led.**

bites, nail punctures: **Hyper., Led.**

injection, from painful: **Hyper.**

lumbar puncture, after: **Hyper.**

palms or soles, of: **Hyper., Led.**

RAPE victims: **Acon., Arn., Ign., Staph.**

SCIATICA: *Coloc.,* **Hyper.,** *Phyt., Rhus-t.*

SHINGLES:

acute attack: **Ran–b., Rhus–t.**

postzonal neuralgia: **Mez.**

SHOULDER injury: *Arn., Bry.,* **Rhus–t.**

SPRAINS: Arn., Bry., Rhus–t., Ruta

ankles or knees, of: **Led., Rhus–t., Ruta**

shoulder: **Rhus–t.**

wrists: **Rhus–t., Ruta**

STINGS, insects from: **Apis,** *Bell., Calad.,*
Hyper., Led., Urt–u.

bee: **Apis, Carb–ac.**

jellyfish: **Apis,** Hyper., Urt–u.

wasp: **Apis**

yellow jacket: **Led.**

STRAIN, from overexertion: **Arn., Rhus–t.,
Ruta**

STROKE, acute or recent: **Arn.**

SUNSTROKE: Bell., Glon., Sol.

SURGERY, complications from:

anesthesia, problems from: **Phos.**

bleeding, after: **Phos.**

healing, to promote, after: **Calen.**

trauma, bruises to tissues: **Arn.**

wounds, of: **Calen.**★

TEA, indisposition from drinking: **Chin., Puls.**

TEETH:

abscess of: **Hep., Sil.**

extraction, bleeding after: **Phos.**

pain after: **Arn.**

filling, pain after: **Arn.**

nerve, exposed: **Cham.**

TENDONS, injuries to: Arn., **Rhus-t., Ruta**

TOENAIL, ingrown: **Sil.**

THRUSH: Bor.

VACCINATIONS, acute reactions to: **Hyper., Led., Sil.**

after-effects from: **Led., Sil.**

VOMITING: Ars., Colch., Ip., Nux-v., Tab., Verat.

diarrhea with: **Verat.**

nausea with: **Ars., Colch., Ip.**

nausea not relieved by: **Ip.**

radiation, after: **Cadm.,** *Ip.*

WRIST injuries: **Hyper., Ruta**

WRITER'S cramp: **Mag-p.**

★*Note:* Before surgery, take Phosphorus 200C 3 pellets, dry in the mouth, to protect yourself against the anesthesia and to stop the bleeding. Afterwards, use Calendula to heal the incision and Arnica to reduce bruising, swelling and pain. For each remedy, dissolve one pellet of 200C in 4 oz. of water, (using separate cups for each) and sip as needed.

Coughs and Colds

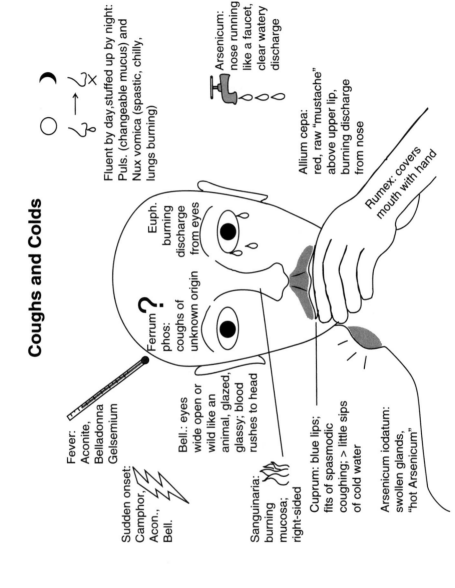

Fever:
Aconite,
Belladonna
Gelsemium

Sudden onset:
Camphor.,
Acon.,
Bell.

Ferrum phos: coughs of unknown origin

Bell.: eyes wide open or wild like an animal, glazed, glassy; blood rushes to head

Sanguinaria: burning mucosa; right-sided

Euph. burning discharge from eyes

Fluent by day, stuffed up by night: Puls. (changeable mucus) and Nux vomica (spastic, chilly, lungs burning)

Arsenicum: nose running like a faucet, clear watery discharge

Allium cepa: red, raw "mustache" above upper lip, burning discharge from nose

Rumex: covers mouth with hand

Cuprum: blue lips; fits of spasmodic coughing; > little sips of cold water

Arsenicum iodatum: swollen glands, "hot Arsenicum"

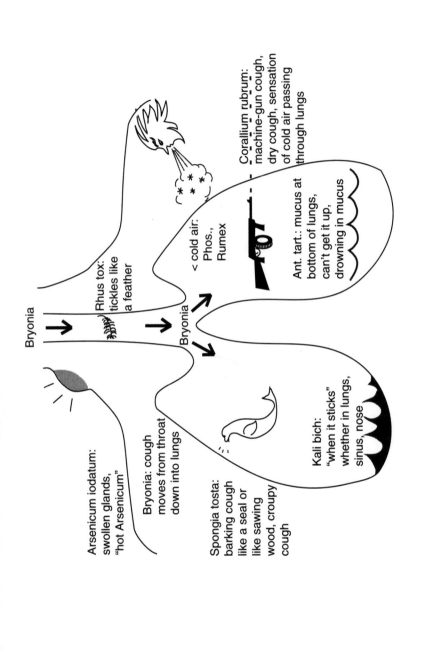

Arsenicum iodatum: swollen glands, "hot Arsenicum"

Rhus tox: tickles like a feather

Bryonia

Bryonia: cough moves from throat down into lungs

Bryonia

< cold air: Phos., Rumex

Corallium rubrum: machine-gun cough, dry cough, sensation of cold air passing through lungs

Ant. tart.: mucus at bottom of lungs, can't get it up, drowning in mucus

Spongia tosta: barking cough like a seal or like sawing wood, croupy cough

Kali bich: "when it sticks" whether in lungs, sinus, nose

Coughs, Colds and Flus

COUGH

AIR:

< cold: **Hep., Phos., Rumex**

< dry, cold: **Acon., Hep.**

< going from warm to cold: *Phos.*, **Rumex**

BARKING (like a seal): **Acon., Bell., Dros., Hep., Spong.**

CHICKEN-POX, after: Ant-c.

CHOKING: Alum., Coc-c., Hep., **Ip.,** *Kali-bi., Lach.*

sleep, as soon as one falls asleep: **Lach.**

COLD drinks:

< **Ars.,** *Phos., Spong.*

> **Caust., Cupr.**

CROUPY: Acon., Hep., Kali-bi., Phos., *Rumex,* **Samb., Spong.**

wheezing and suffocation, with: **Samb.**

DEEP enough, sensation as though he could not cough, to start mucus: **Caust.**

DISTRESSING: Caust., Nux-v.

DRY: Acon., Alum., Ars., Bell., Bry., Hep., Nux-v., Phos., Puls., Rumex, Spong.

daytime: **Spong.**

evening: **Hep.,** *Nux-v.,* **Puls.,** *Spong.,* **Sulph.**

night: **Ars., Bell., Dros., Hep., Phos., Puls., Spong., Sulph.**

DRY cough at night, *continued:*

    < lying: *Puls.*, **Sulph.**

    > sitting up: Puls.

    waking from sleep: Puls., **Sulph.**

      > drinking: *Caust.*, **Spong.**

    expectoration only in a.m.: Bry., Phos., **Puls.**

    menses, before: *Sulph.*, **Zinc.**

    sleep, during: **Cham.**, *Rhus-t.*

    tickling in larynx, from: **Lyc.**, **Puls.**

EXERTION: *Lyc.*, *Nux-v.*, **Puls.**

EXHAUSTING: Ars., **Bell.**, **Caust.**, *Cupr.*,

    Nux-v., *Phos.*, **Stann.**

    night: *Caust.*, **Puls.**

    sleep, disturbing: **Puls.**

INABILITY to: *Dros.*

    > pressure of hand on stomach: *Dros.*

LOOSE: Ars., *Dulc.*, *Phos.*, **Puls.**, *Stann.*

MUCUS, chest, in: **Kali-bi.**, **Puls.**, **Stann.**

    throat, in: *Cupr.*, **Kali-bi.**, **Lach.**, *Nux-v.*

PERSISTENT: Bell., **Cupr.**, *Nux-v.*

    day and night: **Spong.**

    < lying on back, > on side: *Nux-v.*

PREGNANCY, during: *Caust.*

RATTLING: Ant-t., **Caust.**, **Ip.**, *Kali-bi.*, **Puls.**,

    Sulph.

    chest, in, difficult to bring up: **Ant-t.**

SIT UP, must: *Ars.*, *Bry.*, *Kali-bi.*, **Phos.**, **Puls.**,

    Samb.

SLEEP, preventing: Kali-bi., **Lyc.**, **Puls.**, *Rhus-t.*

**SUFFOCATING: Alum., Carb-v., Dros.,
Hep., Ip., Nux-v., Samb., Sulph.**

  night: **Ars.,** *Carb-v., Cupr.*

  child becomes blue in face: *Cupr.,* **Ip.**

TALKING, inability to speak, with: *Cupr., Rumex*

TICKLING: Acon., Cham., Ip., *Kali-bi.,*
Nux-v., *Phos., Puls., Rhus-t., Rumex, Spong.*

  air, in open: **Phos.**

  chest: *Kali-bi., Nux-v.,* **Phos., Stann.**

  throat, from: **All-c., Ars., Bell., Coc-c.,
  Dros., Ip., Nux-c., Phos., Puls., Spong.**

UNCOVERING agg: Hep., Rhus-t., Rumex

  feet or head: **Sil.**

WARM drinks amel.: **Ars., Lyc., Nux-v., Rhus-
t., Sil.,** *Spong.*

WHOOPING: *Bry.,* **Carb-v., Dros.,** *Kali-bi.,
Phos., Puls., Rumex, Spong.*

WIND, in the: *Acon.,* **Hep.**

EXPECTORATION

DIFFICULT: Caust., Ip., Puls.
　sticking to throat: **Kali-bi.**
GREYISH: Lyc., Stann.
GREENISH: Carb-v., Kali-bi., Lyc., Merc.,
　Nat-s., Phos., Puls., Stann., Sulph.
ROPY (stringy): **Kali-bi.**
THICK: Hep., Hydr., Kali-bi., *Puls.,* **Sil.,**
　Stann.
　morning: *Phos., Puls.,* **Stann.**
WHITE: Lyc., Phos., *Puls., Spong., Stann., Sulph.*
YELLOW: Hep., Hydr., Lyc., Phos., Puls.,
　Sil., *Spong.,* **Stann.**

COLDS

DISCHARGE:
　burning: **All-c.,** *Ars.,* **Puls.,** *Merc., Phos., Sil.,*
　　Sulph.
　clear, watery: **Ars.**
　eggwhite, like: **Nat-m.**
　green: **Kali-bi., Puls.**
　raw, makes skin under nose raw: **Al-c.**
　variable: **Puls.**
　yellow: **Puls.**
DRYNESS inside the nose: **Ars., Bell., Carb-v.,**
　Caust., **Kali-bi., Lyc., Phos., Samb., Sulph.**
　blowing nose, compelled, but no discharge:
　　Kali-bi.

65

ITCHING of the nose: **Arum-t., Caust., Cina,**
Lyc., Merc., Nux-v., **Sulph.**

MUCUS PLUGS in nose:

crusts, scabs inside nose: *Ars.,* **Kali-bi.**, *Nux-v.,*
Rhus-t.

hard to detach: **Kali-bi.**

re-form if detach: **Kali-bi.**

elastic plugs: **Kali-bi.**

green masses: **Kali-bi.**

NOSE, RUNNY: **Ars., Kali-bi., Lyc., Merc.,**
Nux-v., Puls., Sil.

air, from a draft of: *Dulc., Merc.*

air, in open amel.: **Puls.**

chilliness, with: *Ars.,* **Merc., Nux-v.**

chilled, from becoming chilled while over-
heated: **Ars.**

discharge, with (see also **DISCHARGE**):

daytime: **Nux-v.**

morning: **Nux-v.**

after rising: **Nux-v.**

in open air: **Nit-ac., Puls.**

in warm room: **All-c., Puls.**

extends to sinuses (sinusitis): *Kali-bi.,* **Lyc.,**
Merc., *Puls.,* **Sil.**

< evening: **All-c.**

hayfever: **All-c., Ambr.,** *Euphr., Puls.,* **Sabad.**

left-sided: **Arum-t.**

< morning: **Nux-v.**

< night: **Merc.**

postnasal drip: **Hep.**, *Hydr.*, **Kali-bi.**, *Sil.*

right-sided: **Ars.**, **Nux-v.**

SNEEZING:
frequent: **Ars.**, **Carb-v.**, **Coc-c.**, **Merc.**,
    Nux-v., **Sulph.**

sleep during: *Puls.*

warm room, in: **Puls.**

THROAT

DISCOLORATION (color of throat):
purple: **Lach.**, *Puls.*

red: **Acon.**, *Apis,* **Bell.**, **Caps.**, **Lyc.**, **Phyt.**,
    Sulph.

tonsils red: **Bell.**, *Merc.*

white: *Mur-ac.*, **Nit-ac.**

INFLAMMATION (sore):
right side: **Ars.**, **Bell.**, **Lyc.**, *Merc.*, **Phyt.**

left side: *Hep.*, **Lach.**, *Nit-ac.*

whole throat: **Apis, Ferr-p.**, **Merc.**

night at: **Merc.**

PAIN (see inflammation):
cold drinks amel.: **Phyt.**

warm drinks amel.: **Ars.**, **Hep.**, **Lyc.**, *Sulph.*

extending to ear: *Bell.*, *Hep.*, *Lach.*, **Nit-ac.**,
    Nux-v.

SWALLOWING:
fluids, can only swallow fluids: *Bapt.*, *Sil.*

fluids agg.: **Lach.**, *Merc.*

more difficult than solids: **Lach.**

FLU

COMMON remedies: *Arn.,* **Ars.,** *Bapt., Bry.,*
Eup-per., Gels., *Ip., Rhus-t.*
bones ache: **Eup-per.**
chilly, restless: **Ars.**
damp weather, worse in: **Rhus-t.**
diarrhea, vomiting, with: **Bapt.**
trembling and exhaustion, with: **Gels.**
PREVENTION: Ars., Oscillococcinum
SUMMER flu (diarrhea, vomiting): **Ars., Ip.,
Nux-v.**
POST-INFLUENZA COMPLICATIONS:
cough: **Sulph.**
fatigue: **China-a., Kali-p.**

Flu

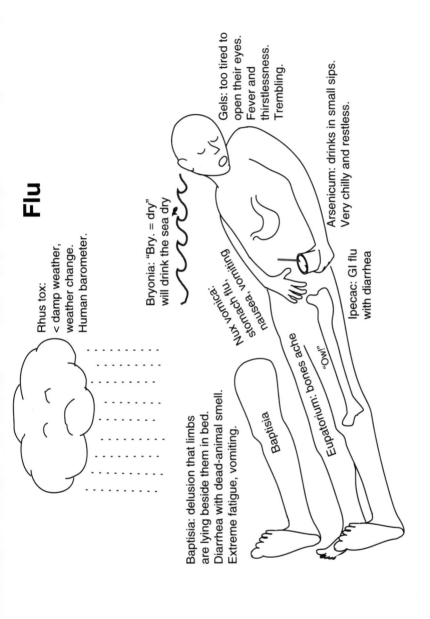

Rhus tox:
< damp weather,
weather change.
Human barometer.

Gels: too tired to
open their eyes.
Fever and
thirstlessness.
Trembling.

Bryonia: "Bry. = dry"
will drink the sea dry

Arsenicum: drinks in small sips.
Very chilly and restless.

Nux vomica:
stomach flu,
nausea, vomiting

Ipecac: GI flu
with diarrhea

Baptisia: delusion that limbs
are lying beside them in bed.
Diarrhea with dead-animal smell.
Extreme fatigue, vomiting.

Eupatorium: bones ache
"Ow!"

Baptisia

Women's Health

WARNING: remedies should only be taken after a gyne-cological exam and in cooperation with your gynecologist!

PREGNANCY, LABOR and NURSING

Pregnancy, during:
    constipation: **Nux-v.**
    discharge: **Sep.**
    headaches: **Sep.**
    incontinence of urine: **Puls.**
    vaginal itching: **Calad.**
    varicose veins: **Puls.**
    vertigo: **Nat-m.**
Morning sickness (nausea in pregnancy): **Colch.,**
    Ip., *Phos.,* **Sep.**
    morning, in bed: **Nux-v.**
        on rising: *Nux-v., Sep.*
    breakfast, before: **Sep.**
    deathly nausea: **Ip.**
    eggs, smell of, after: **Colch.**
    fish, smell of, after: **Colch.**
    food, looking at: **Colch.**
        smell of: **Colch.**
        thought of: **Colch.**
    putting hands in warm water: **Phos.**
    vomiting: **Ip., Phos., Sep.**
Before childbirth:
    fear: **Acon., Gels.**

contractions, to prepare for: **Caul.** (see specific directions under Caulophyllum in the *Guide to the Remedies*)

During childbirth:

cessation (stopping) of contractions: *Cimic., Gels.*

dilate cervix: **Cimic.**

faintness during labor: **Puls.**

impatience with: **Cham.**

legs, cramping in the, with: **Cupr., Mag-p.**

nausea, with: **Ip.**

pain in back: **Gels., Nux-v.**

painful contractions: *Bell.,* **Cham.,** *Mag-p.*

bear the pains, can hardly: **Cham.**

weeping: **Puls.**

After childbirth

after-pains: **Cham., Sep.**

depression ("postpartum blues"): **Sep.**

episiotomy, to heal: **Calen.**

hair loss, ongoing: **Lach.**

trauma/bruising: **Arn., Bell-p.**

urine, retention of (absence of): **Caust., Puls.**

weakness, exhaustion: **Kali-p.**

Breastfeeding:

inflammation of the breast during: **Phyt.**

milk production, to stimulate: **Lac-d.**

to stop: **Lac-c.**

suppressed from grief: **Ign.**

nipples, sore: **Arn., Nux-v., Sulph.**

BREASTFEEDING, *continued:*
    cracked: **Graph., Sulph.**
    weakness from nursing: **Chin.**

PMS and MENSTRUATION

MENSTRUAL CRAMPS: Bell., Cham., *Coff.,*
Coloc., Mag-p., Puls.
    > double bent over: **Mag-p.**
    heaviness, feeling of: **Puls.**
    labor-like pains: **Cham.**
    nausea, with: **Nux-v.**
    nervous excitement, with: **Coff.**
    painful: **Cact., Cham., Mag-p.**

MENSES, suppressed (stopped) from:
    anger: **Coloc.**
    cold or chill due to dampness: **Puls.**
    feet wet and chilled, from becoming: **Puls.**
    fright: *Acon.*
    grief: **Ign.**
    wet and chilled, from becoming: **Rhus-t.**

PMS:
    anger and irritability: **Sep.**
    fatigue: **Sep.**
    insomnia: **Sep.**
    water retention: **Apis**
    weepiness, depression: **Sep.**

Note: menopause is not covered here because it requires professional homeopathic treatment.

OTHER CONDITIONS

BREAST, inflammation of (mastitis): **Bell., Bry., Phyt.**

with stitching pains (sensation of a needle pricking): **Bry.**

DISCHARGE (leucorrhea):

burning: **Kreos., Puls., Sulph.**

cottage cheese-like: *Hep.*

cream-like: **Puls.**

girls, in little: *Puls.,* **Sep.**

intercourse, after: *Sep.*

yellow: **Hydr., Sep., Sulph.**

white: **Graph., Sep.**

HONEYMOON CYSTITIS: Staph.

ITCHING, vaginal: **Calad., Kreos., Nit-ac., Sep.**

evening: *Kreos.*

intense, voluptuous: **Kreos.**

intercourse, after: **Nit-ac.**

MISCARRIAGE or ABORTION, after:

bruising of birth canal: **Bell-p.**

grief: **Ignatia**

toning of uterus: **Bell-p.**

weakness: **China**

PAIN, in ovaries:

right-sided: **Apis, Bell.**

left-sided: **Coloc.**

PAIN, vaginal:

burning: **Nit-ac., Sulph.**

preventing coition: **Cact.**

RAPE, sexual abuse:
    suppressed anger, humiliation: **Staph.**
    bruising: **Arn.**
    emotional trauma: **Staph.**
    fright, shock: **Acon.**
VAGINITIS (inflammation of vagina):
    itching and burning: **Sulph.**
    itching and soreness: **Caust.**
    itching and stinging: **Apis**

PART FOUR

A Guide
to the Remedies

Once you have found your remedy in the Repertory, you can learn more about it in this section. And if you have found several possible remedies in the Repertory, this section will help you decide between them. Striking characteristics of the remedies (called "keynotes") are in **bold.** *The remedy names in this section are the ones we use when talking about the remedies, rather than the short abbreviations in the Repertory (Ferrum phos. for example, not Ferr-p, or Nat. mur. instead of Nat-m.)*

Aconitum napellus *(monkshood)*

Aconite stands for the **4 F's:** Fast–Fever–Fulminant–Fright. 'Fast', because it belongs to an acute, sudden-onset illness. For instance, the child goes to bed peacefully and wakes up around **midnight** with sudden **high fever (104°-105° F),** restless and full of **fear,** screaming for his mother. He feels **very hot all over the body** and is **very thirsty** for large quantities of cold water. The word 'fulminant' relates to the high fever. Aconite has a strong disease picture, "as if a storm started suddenly in the patient." This typically happens when the child has played outside in a cold, dry wind as often happens in the winter. The child gets sweaty, throws his jacket off, and gets chilled.

Aconite is most often used for sore throats, beginning cold with dry hacking cough, conjunctivitis, pharyngitis, sudden fright (almost got killed in an accident, after an earthquake, any other shock situation; it has been called the homeopathic "Valium").

Agaricus muscarius *(crazy mushroom)*

Agaricus is the number one remedy for **twitching**. For the purpose of this book, its main indication is in **frostbite**. It should be part of the homeopathic rescue kit of any mountaineer. A sign you should use Agaricus is the presence of cold spots, especially in the feet, or a sensation of cold or hot needles.

Allium cepa *(red onion)*

All of us who have cut an onion know what effect the onion has on us: **bland** (non-irritating) **tearing of the eyes,** with a runny nose **(burning and acrid).** The running of the nose peels away (excoriates) the skin under the nose where the watery discharge occurs. At the same time there is severe sneezing.

Allium cepa is most often used for an acute attack of **hayfever.** Note that it has exactly the **opposite** symptoms of **Euphrasia,** another acute hayfever remedy. Any allergy attack which has the above symptoms (sneezing, nose running and chapping the upper lip) will respond well to this remedy.

A little known use is for the treatment of acute pain in an amputated limb **(neuralgia of the phantom limb)**: the patient complaints of pain in the missing limb, hence the name "phantom."

Alumina *(aluminum)*

The main action of this metal is on the nervous system. The reader may be familiar with the possible link between Alzheimer's disease and the use of aluminum pots and pans for cooking. And indeed, in the provings of Alumina, memory loss has been noted (as though the brain has dried up) as well as slowness in answering questions. This indicates that Alumina may well be a good remedy for some patients with Alzheimer's.

For household use, Alumina is useful in severe cases of **constipation** where the person has no urge to go or has to strain a lot with very little result. A special symptom is that he feels **worse from eating potatoes.**

Anacardium orientale *(marking nut)*

This interesting remedy—which has its chronic use for some forms of Tourette's syndrome as well as for split personalities—is important to us here for its power to rapidly alleviate the effects of **poison oak and poison ivy.** It can also relieve **headaches in students** (like Calc. phos.).

Antimonium tartaricum *(tartar emetic)*

Ant. tart. has a great action on the respiratory system since it corresponds to a great **rattling of mucus in the chest, difficult to bring up.** More and more children in this country are little "mucus producers." (For an explanation of why asthma and excessive mucus production in children have become so widespread in this generation, see my book *Human Condition: Critical*). The child has difficulties breathing because of the abundance of thick, white mucus in the chest which can be heard from a distance (difficult, noisy breathing with shortness of breath).

Ant. tart. is also one of the top remedies for **whooping cough and chickenpox.**

Apis mellifica *(honeybee, queen bee)*

If you have been stung by a bee, then you know when to use this remedy: there is a **stinging, burning** pain, a **swelling** locally, and a **redness**. Whenever you see these symptoms anywhere in the body (throat or knee or other joints), Apis is indicated. The area of swelling is **worse from cold** (for example, worse from applying an ice pack) and feels better from warmth. The person **desires open air** and has *no* **thirst**.

Apis has many acute indications: hives (urticaria), especially after eating shellfish and strawberries; acute sore throat with the above characteristic symptoms; insect bites (it is the top remedy for wasp and ant bites); PMS with water retention; and joint pains with stinging, burning pains and swelling.

Argentum nitricum *(silver nitrate)*

Argentum nitricum is called the **"What if"** remedy: the person is full of **anticipation anxiety**. He is anxious about an upcoming test, an interview, an audition, always anticipating the worst. These people are always hurrying, driven, excitable, hyper and in a state of worry, which easily leads to **diarrhea** and palpitations, to the point that they hate going to public places. Thus this remedy is greatly indicated for stage fright, examination funk, and fear of public speaking.

People who need Argentum nitricum typically have an intense craving for sweets, salt and chocolate.

Silver nitrate is put in the eyes of every newborn (unfortunately not in homeopathic doses) to avoid the possibility of gonorrhea being transmitted from the mother. It is therefore also indicated in conjunctivitis with yellow/green discharge. Another indication is colic in babies. It is the number one remedy for this common destroyer of the new mother's sleep!

Arnica montana *(leopard's bane, a mountain daisy)*

Arnica is called the **sports** remedy for its great indications in sports traumas when there is a typical **sore, bruised** feeling, with the impression "that a truck drove over me." Pains are **worse by the slightest touch** (so that the person is afraid of being touched) and better from cold applications.

Arnica is indicated in **any blunt trauma** where the skin is not opened. (Use Calendula when the skin is broken as it will speed healing faster, and Arnica may actually be harmful in this situation.) Arnica is especially useful to absorb blood under the skin (hematomas). It is also good for the trauma after childbirth, post-operatively, for overlifting (moving furniture, working in the yard), overexertion of muscles (especially when you haven't used them for a while), falls, accidents where the person can be in shock, and even overuse of the voice (strained voice). It should be given to any acute **stroke** victim as it absorbs internal bleeding very quickly, therefore limiting the damage of bleeding (when bleeding is the cause of the stroke). It is also an excellent **flu** remedy when the typical sore, bruised feeling is present.

Arsenicum album *(arsenic)*

Yes, the greatest poisons make the best remedies, as long as they are administered in a homeopathic dose. Arsenicum is one of the most widely used homeopathic remedies. You should "never leave home without it" as it is the best indicated remedy for **food poisoning.** The diarrhea and vomiting are quickly relieved and no further consequences are expected. Always travel with Arsenicum album!

People who need Arsenicum are often very restless individuals, anxious and often labeled "hypochondriacs" as they always seem to be searching for a disease. An Arsenicum state is one of great restlessness, with extreme fatigue and severe anxiety. Therefore it is often used acutely in a **severe asthma attack**, especially for an attack between 1-3 a.m., in which the person has to get out of bed to relieve his shortness of breath and severe wheezing. These people typically require an extra pillow for sleeping to make breathing easier and are thirsty for small sips of cold water. There is often a **periodicity** (regular recurrence) to these asthma attacks: every two days, every three days, every seven days, etc.

Besides its uses for food poisoning and asthma, Arsenicum is the first remedy to think of for any **beginning cold** with a clear, runny nose (with or without relentless sneezing or a right-sided sore throat). It is a great **flu** remedy (a universal one) which can also be used for flu prevention (a 200C dose, 3 pellets dry, once a week during the flu season).

No remedy brings more relief to the **dying patient** than Arsenicum in a 200C potency: it calms the struggling patient without doping him. He stays alert yet not anxious, which is a relief for the family and patient alike. The picture of a dying patient wanting to hang onto life is not a pretty one, and can cause additional anguish to the family in their time of grief.

Aurum metallicum *(the metal gold)*

The main idea of this remedy is **depression** and loathing of life, to the point that people who need Aurum chronically want to commit suicide (by jumping out of a window). They are usually very ambitious people who pressure themselves with the greatest expectations (students who want to be first in their class, business people who "put all their eggs in one basket" like in the stockmarket). Whenever life does not pan out as they have planned, life has no meaning for them anymore and they become depressed. The same situation can occur when a teenager who is a good student gets depressed because he cannot go to the college of his dreams, due to financial problems in the family. As one can see, this remedy is often related to financial matters, as one would expect from the remedy gold.

Another situation in which Aurum has great value is when one of the two partners in a long-time marriage dies: the surviving partner feels that life is not worth living anymore. "I have lost the sunshine of my life," they claim and not uncommonly, they die shortly after the death of their partner. So many people in nursing homes could use this remedy as they are often in a state of **"abandonment"**: no more spouse or husband, few friends left in their life, and often few visits from other family members. These people could truly say that the sunshine has gone from their lives. In fact for many traditional cultures the metal gold (Aurum) is associated with the sun.

Baptisia tinctoria *(wild indigo)*

Baptisia was *the* **flu** remedy of the infamous Spanish flu pandemic (worldwide epidemic) of 1918, in which at least 200,000 Americans died. However, according to records preserved in English hospitals, the death rate in homeopathic hospitals was less than 5%, while the death rate in conventional hospitals with Western medicine was 45% (a triumph for homeo–

pathy which Western medicine should take notice of)!

Baptisia is a typical flu remedy, but not usually one of the top ones (except in 1918). The symptoms are extreme tiredness, mental confusion, high fever with **extreme bad odor of all discharges and secretions** (stool, urine, perspiration, breath, etc.). At the height of the illness, the person suffers from **delusions** in which he thinks that his leg is lying next to him in bed (extremities separated from the body). The person is in a **stupor** state, "as if he is drunk."

Belladonna *(deadly nightshade)*

One derivative of this plant is atropine, used in Western medicine. This "poison" is well-known for its use in **acute febrile conditions: sudden** onset of symptoms ("as if a storm was aroused in the person") and intense **redness** and **heat of the face** ("as if all the blood of the body was pooled in the face") with **cold extremities**. The eyes are wide open with dilated pupils; the person can have a wild animal-like look and a sensation of **throbbing, pulsating** pains. The symptoms end as suddenly as they began; they are typically worst around **3 p.m.** and 9 p.m., and are worse from noise, jarring, **light** (extreme sensitivity to bright light!), **high temperatures** (103°-104° F) with possible delirium and hallucinations, dry mouth but not a great thirst!

Note: the person who needs Arsenicum is thirsty for little sips of cold water; one who needs Aconite is thirsty for cold drinks; and one who needs Gelsemium is thirstless. Belladonna is a **right-sided** remedy (i.e. symptoms such as a sore throat or headache tend to occur on the right side).

Belladonna is indicated in all conditions showing the above symptoms: **sore throats**, flus, early stages of abscesses and **ear infections**. It can prevent convulsions associated with high fever in children. In the past it was used for rabies.

Bellis perennis *(English daisy)*

Another treasure of our garden. It should be routinely given after childbirth as it has a great affinity for the female pelvic area. A 200C dose right after childbirth is extremely healing for the trauma and bruising of the birth canal. It also brings back the muscle tone of the uterus. It is also called the "gardener's remedy" as it is a deeper-working remedy than Arnica, indicated in all kind of traumas where Arnica does not completely heal, and in rheumatism. It is a very specific remedy for tennis elbow, the great fear of tennis players (Ruta is another good remedy). It is also very specific for any blunt trauma to the breast and can be used after mammography if the breasts are painful or bruised from the procedure.

Berberis vulgaris *(barberry)*

Berberis is most useful for an **acute attack from kidney stones**, especially if the pain is located on the left side, typically radiating from the kidney and extending to the bladder with spastic pains.

Bryonia *(wild hops)*

There is probably no remedy better known for **headaches** than Bryonia. It is called for in headaches or other acute pain syndromes (like from injury) which are **worse from the slightest movement.** Typically the person has the flu with a severe headache and they want to be left alone, in the dark, with no noise—to the point they don't want to speak for fear of making their headache worse. Even opening their eyes would aggravate their headache!

Bryonia is typically used for the headache which **starts above the left eye,** goes to the back of the head and then engulfs the whole head. It is an acute, piercing pain, **worse at 9 p.m.** The onset is **gradual** (unlike the sudden onset of Belladonna), and the headache feels better from local applications of heat. There is **improvement** of the pain with **strong pressure or lying on the painful side** as it prevents the motion of that part. The person is **very thirsty** (feels as though he "could drink the sea dry!") and he has a very dry mouth; in fact all the mucous membranes are dry.

Bryonia is useful for all **fever conditions** in which we see the above symptoms (especially ones in which the person does not want to move!). It works well for colds beginning in the nose and going down to the chest. From there it is a great remedy for avoiding and treating **pneumonia** and pleurisy. It is also good for acute rheumatic conditions with shooting pains, again with the typical aggravation from the slightest movement.

Bryonia is also called for in cases of **constipation** in which the person has no desire for stool; when the stools finally come, they are dry, hard, and painful to expel. It is also a **great pain remedy** for whiplash and broken bones (as are Arnica, which reduces swelling and resorbs blood under the skin, and Symphytum, which helps to repair the broken bones).

Calendula officinalis *(garden marigold)*

Calendula should be available in every household since it is known for its great healing qualities in cuts and abrasions. It should be routinely used after every operation or dental work (whenever the skin is cut or broken), as it acts both as an antiseptic (to prevent infection) and as a healing agent. It promotes healing so fast that a dentist friend of mine claims he can see the granulation (wound healing process) take place before his very eyes during dental surgery. Indeed, Calendula will control bleeding from open wounds.

Just remember, use *only* Calendula on open wounds, *never* Arnica!

Calendula is also used for second and third degree burns, and—like Phosphorus and Millefolia—for bleeding situations such as bleeding gums, ruptured eardrums, and nosebleeds. It is available in cream form like Arnica, but the action of these remedies is speedier and deeper when the pellets are dissolved in water and taken orally.

Cantharis *(Spanish fly)*

Cantharis is a specific remedy for **bladder infections** where there is a **burning pain, before, during and even after** urination. When a urine culture has been taken, Cantharis will often take the pain away and cure the whole process before the results even come back from the lab. The pains are violent, sharp and burning, and blood may even be seen in the urine.

Cantharis is also the best remedy for second degree burns and sunburns with blister formation.

Capsicum *(red or chili pepper)*

And you thought your kitchen ingredients were only for cooking! Many of our seasonings are proven as homeopathic remedies (Natrum muriaticum, table salt, is one of our best known remedies). There are two main uses for Capsicum which have nothing to do with each other. One is for **acute sore throats** with the sensation **"as if a hot pepper is put on the tongue."** The other is for cases of **homesickness**. No remedy works better than Capsicum for the nostalgic, homesick summer camper or college student away from home for the first time.

Carbo vegetalis *(charcoal)*

The main idea of Carbo veg. is **lack of oxygen.**You can see the person sitting on a chair, gasping for air, fanning himself or wanting a fan to be directed at him (he desires air!); he feels cold and may be belching and passing gas. Not a pretty sight! The person may look as though he is going to die anytime.

Carbo veg. can be a life-saver in **asthma attacks** or any other conditions with shortness of breath (let your homeopathic physician decide this). More practical for the layperson is its use in **digestive disturbances** in which there is severe **bloating above** the navel (Lycopodium is for bloating under the navel, China for the whole abdomen bloating). **Belching** and **passing gas** accompany the bloating.

Carbo veg. is lesser known but of great value for **altitude sickness.** Many people complain of headaches, shortness of breath, palpitations, etc. when they visit high altitude locations like Colorado or New Mexico. Apparently the Colorado Chamber of Commerce is concerned about this issue, as tourism is a great source of income for the state. Carbo veg. is their solution. It goes without saying that Carbo veg., along with Agaricus, should be in every mountaineer's emergency kit!

Carbo veg. will also help stop postpartum bleeding following abortions.

Carbolic acid *(phenol)*

Carbolic acid is the #1 remedy for beestings and great for allergic reactions to them. Acutely we also use it for burns which tend to ulcerate. Conditions which require Carbolic acid are characterized by terrible, burning and pricking pains, with a sensation of pricking like needles. In the past it was also used for the fatigue lingering from a flu, and for destructive conditions in general causing severe fatigue.

Caulophyllum *(blue cohosh)*

Those who know the herbal uses of blue cohosh for women's conditions will not be surprised to learn that in homeopathy it is often used professionally in obstetrics and gynecology. It will be mainly used by the layperson (in consultation with her gynecologist) for the **toning of the uterus**. About 3 weeks before the expected date of delivery (not earlier!), start taking Caulophyllum 6c, three pellets dry in the mouth, twice a day. It will ensure strong contractions, shorter labor, and an easy delivery when the baby is due.

Caulophyllum can also be used as a pain remedy in the **rheumatic pains of small joints** (thus more for arthritis or gout in the toes rather than the knees. Use Colchicum for arthritis or gout in the big toe and Caulophyllum for the smaller toes).

Causticum *(potassium hydrate)*

Causticum is mainly used in conditions affecting the central nervous system: the central idea is **paralysis**. This can also mean paralysis of the emotions, as can happen to some unfortunate people who have been subjected to several traumas in a short timespan (loss of friends, children, family in which they act like they can't move, it was just one trauma too much!). In addition to paralysis of the nervous system, Causticum is also used for burning, drawing pains with a feeling that "the tendons are too short."

Causticum can relieve a **stiff neck** (right-sided) and acute carpal tunnel syndrome. It is **predominantly a right-sided** remedy. It is a great remedy for **Bell's palsy** and for **incontinence of urine** in which people lose urine when they are running, coughing, laughing, or sneezing. In these chronic cases, however, you should consult your homeopath.

Clues for using Causticum include symptoms made worse by dry, cold north winds (the person needs a scarf or hat); symptoms worse at 3 a.m.; and symptoms better in a hot, humid climate. (Most people with rheumatism or arthritis feel *worse* in dampness; people with arthritis or rheumatism who feel *better* in dampness almost always need Causticum.) The person who needs Causticum chronically usually has a great sense of justice and great sympathy for others (a child can get tics from seeing another child in a wheelchair, for instance). These people are very sensitive to the wrongs in the world.

Chamomilla *(chamomile flower)*

Chamomilla is a very effective homeopathic remedy for children, but it is much abused in herbal preparations. Who does not know of chamomile for **teething babies**? However, it should be taken in homeopathic doses, as herbal preparations will lead to a proving of the remedy—in other words, a *worsening* of the symptoms. Drinking too much chamomile tea while breastfeeding, or giving too much chamomile to an infant who is crying during teething, can actually create the difficult personality type of the Chamomilla child.

Everyone has met a child of this type: **irritable, quickly angered, fretful, and moody.** They want something, you offer it to them, they throw back to you. They **want to be carried** all the time which seems to be the only way to stop the whining and crying, except for the car ride around the block, which also calms the child. During the teething, the child gets greenish diarrhea "looking like chopped spinach." Symptoms are worse between 9 p.m. and midnight.

The **painkilling** qualities of Chamomilla are also of great benefit in labor pains (in which the woman typically throws the doctor out of the room, cursing him for the pain, yet then calls him back). It also provides effective relief for other unbearable pains such as in dysmenorrhea (painful menses), earache and colic.

Little known but of great benefit is Chamomilla's effect on **coffee withdrawal**. Looking at the symptoms Chamomilla relieves, you can see that it nicely covers the side effects of caffeine withdrawal (even the headaches). Use your Cham. 200C as needed throughout the day; usually after one week the symptoms disappear and you can stop the Cham. (This is a much better solution than one I read about in the newspapers: some doctors now try to protect their patients from caffeine withdrawal after surgery by injecting some coffee into their I.V. lines!)

China officinalis *(cinchona, Peruvian bark)*

This remedy will stay immortal forever, as it was the first remedy proved by Hahnemann. China was to Hahnemann what the falling apple was to Newton. Its active ingredient, quinine, was and still is abused by the medical profession (in the sense that a substance in homeopathic high dilutions will cure a condition which in large drug doses it will cause or intensify; by this standard, quinine in large doses is likely to increase the susceptibilty to, or intensify the symptoms of malaria).

It is sad to think how many people die unnecessarily from malaria. I think about the explorations of Henry Morton Stanley, the Belgian colonist who conquered the present Zaire for the Belgian King Leopold. In spite of huge doses of quinine—or because of it—his porters died by the thousands from malaria. This was nearly a century after Hahnemann proved the effectiveness against malaria of a homeopathic dilution of China. And now we face medication-resistant malaria cases. I predict that China in homeopathic doses will have a great comeback in treating malaria.

China is also an excellent **liver-gallbladder remedy**. Its characteristic symptoms include the **periodicity** (regular recurrence) of symptoms (every other day, every 7th or 14th day); great bloating **all over the abdomen,** with pain not relieved by passing gas; and **painless diarrhea** (especially after eating fruit, but also in food poisoning after eating bad meat). The diarrhea comes gushing out, watery, yellow or colorless accompanied by belching, passing gas, and a bitter taste in the mouth. The abdomen is very sore upon the slightest pressure.

One of the best uses of China is to relieve the pain of a typical **gallbladder attack** due to eating too many rich and fatty foods late at night.

China is also indicated in any situation where there is a **great loss of bodily fluids**: diarrhea, blood loss after operation or miscarriage/abortion, after continuous vomiting, sweating too much as in a sauna, etc. China will restore the bodily weakness in a remarkable way.

Cina *(wormseed)*

Cina was the traditional **worm remedy,** but it was used so much (in large herbal doses) that fatal poisoning often occurred. It was Hahnemann who made it a safe remedy for roundworms and threadworms by diluting it in homeopathic doses.

By the way, there are two "grandmothers' recipes" for expelling worms. To get rid of threadworms, smear the anus with vaseline, inside and out. When the worms come down to breed, they slide out on the lubricant and are gradually passed. Combine this trick with Cina and the worms will be gone for good. My patients can vouch for this method.

The other trick for catching a tapeworm is simple but it works! Tapeworms seem to have a great liking for pumpkin seeds. Shell one ounce of fresh pumpkin seeds, pound them, and mix them with two ounces of honey. Give the mixture to the person in the morning, on an empty stomach, in three doses an hour apart. The tapeworm overeats on the pumpkin seed until it is so relaxed that its hook lets go and it is passed out. Don't touch the worm until it has totally passed, *head and all,* or else the worm will grow again from the head.

How can you tell if your child has worms? Typical symptoms include **grinding the teeth, picking the nose** until it bleeds, biting nails until they bleed, **scratching the anus and ears,** twitching of the eyes, dark circles around the eyes with paleness around the mouth, a **voracious appetite** even immediately after eating, bedwetting, and foul, putrid breath.

The child's behavior is typically **"cross and ugly";** he kicks and hits, wants to be carried all the time, likes to be rocked, is capricious, wants something, then throws it away when he receives it, does not want to be looked at and starts screaming if he is. You have the impression that the child does not know what she wants, except that she wants to be rocked all the time.

Give Cina 200C to these children—it will get rid of the worms and their behavioral problems as well. Cina is highly effective for killing and expelling worms, especially roundworms. Give a single dose of 3 pellets, dry in the mouth, and repeat 7 days later if necessary. It is rarely necessary to repeat a third time.

Cocculus indicus *(Indian cockle tree)*

Western medicine is still looking for a drug which helps people overcome **jet lag** when they travel abroad. Look no further! Cocculus 200C fits the bill perfectly. Take one dose (three pellets dry) when you step on the plane and take another dose when you step off. You might not even need another dose. Do the same thing on your way back. I have done it numerous times myself, and my patients—especially flight attendants—have praised the remedy in these circumstances. It is the #1 remedy for jetlag; other remedies include Arnica, Gelsemium, and Rescue Remedy (a blend of Bach flower remedies).

Other sensations which call for Cocculus include dizziness with exhaustion, which is often seen in **nightwatching**: people taking care of sick or dying relatives for months, always sleeping with one ear open, or loss of sleep after having a baby who cries frequently for the first three months. The person is exhausted, dizzy and emotionally wrecked. I know of no better remedy than Cocculus for this purpose. It is also the #1 remedy for **motion sickness**, especially in the car and airplane (and unlike over-the-counter drugs, it doesn't cause drowsiness!)

Coccus cacti *(cochineal, cactus beetle)*

The main activity of Coccus is on the respiratory mucosa, so it can be used for coughing fits caused by a tickling feeling in the throat, especially around **11:30 p.m.** and in the morning upon awakening. The typical Coccus cough is also made worse by heat, but is relieved when the person is in a cold room or when walking. There is expectoration of **thick, stringy mucus** (similar to Kali bich.). The Coccus cough can be described as a **"machine-gun"** cough: attacks of a spasmodic, rattling cough.

Coffea cruda *(unroasted coffee beans)*

This is the only way Hahnemann would have approved of taking coffee. Think what coffee does to you when you drink it too late at night: you can't sleep because your mind seems to be racing; there is great clarity of mind and abundance of thoughts going through your mind. No wonder it is such a seductive brew! But every action has an equal opposite reaction. Therefore, increasing amounts of coffee are necessary, leading to true addiction (as evidenced by the symptoms of caffeine withdrawal, mentioned under Chamomilla).

So Coffea 200C is indicated in **sleeplessness** created by overjoyous events or **pleasant surprises** (winning the lottery, falling in love with someone new, upcoming marriage, etc.). Who said that joy and happy feelings could not be hazardous to your health?

Other indications are **toothache** (also Hypericum) relieved by cold water, and **headaches** with a feeling "as if a nail has been pounded in the side of your head." Coffea can be used for coffee headache withdrawals but Chamomilla is a better remedy for this.

Colchicum autumnale *(meadow saffron)*

There are two great acute indications for Colchicum: first, for **morning sickness** when the pregnant woman is especially sensitive to odors. The woman gets nauseated at the sight, smell, and even the thought of food, especially the smell of eggs.

The other indication for Colchicum is an **acute attack of gout** in the big toe where the person cannot tolerate the slightest touch or movement (Ledum and Urtica urens are also effective in this situation. Use Caulophyllum for gout or arthritis in the smaller toes.).

Colocynthis *(bitter apple, bitter cucumber)*

Colocynth is another great pain remedy, indicated for pains following a humiliation with suppressed anger. The physical body reacts with a **violent, cutting, stabbing and pinching pain**, especially in the digestive tract or **abdomen**. The pain is relieved by strong pressure and heat, and by **doubling up or bending forward**. It is usually located on the left side. (If pain with the same qualities occurs on the right side, think about Mag. phos.)

Colocynth is also indicated in **menstrual pains** with the above symptoms, for left-sided functional ovary pain, and for **left-sided sciatica** (Hypericum is also good for this).

Cuprum metallicum *(the metal copper)*

Cuprum is for any spasmodic pain that **begins and ends suddenly**. It is one of the greatest **anti-spasmodic** painkillers. The convulsive spasms (anywhere in the body—stomach, abdomen, chest, or a spasmodic cough) are so strong that the person clenches his fist while the face can be blue. Cuprum is a great help for those unbearable, dry, whooping-like coughs which **improve only by drinking small sips of cold water**. It is also a great help for severe **cramps in the calves** (charley horses) in elderly people at night.

Drosera rotundifolia *(sundew plant)*

Drosera was the main remedy Hahnemann used for **whooping cough**. Indeed a **dry, barking, croupy cough** responds well to Drosera. There is an oppression in the chest and the pain is only relieved by exerting great pressure on the chest with both hands. The bouts of coughing occur close to each other so that the person hardly has the time to take a breath. At the end of such an attack, there is often **vomiting**. The cough is **worse after midnight**, worse when lying down, and worse from the heat of the bed.

Drosera also helps to relieve speaker's sore throat (as do Rhus tox. and Arnica).

Eupatorium perfoliatum *(boneset or agueweed)*

Eupatorium is one of the greatest **flu** remedies when the main symptom is pain in the **bones** instead of the muscles. There is fever with bone aches, "**as if the bones would break.**" There is also outspoken **stiffness** of the whole body, with a bruised feeling (Arnica), restlessness and intense thirst for cold water (Aconite).

Equisetum hiemale *(horsetail)*

Equisetum has a great action on the urinary tract where it is especially helpful for **bedwetting** in children. Either prescribe the 6C daily or order the tincture from your health food store. If using the tincture, give 10 drops twice a day in 1 oz. of water (in this case drinking all the water at once).

Euphrasia *(eyebright)*

Its common name, "eyebright," says it all: Euphrasia is a great **eye** remedy, especially for conjunctivitis with violent attacks of profuse secretion of **hot, irritating tears** with **non-irritating nose secretion** (see Allium cepa, which has the opposite types of discharge). These symptoms also correspond to some of the typical **hayfever** attacks. So allergic hayfever, stinging eyes, and dust or sand in the eyes are all good uses for eyebright.

Ferrum phosphoricum *(iron phosphate)*

One of the twelve tissue salts introduced by Schuessler, Ferrum phos. is one of the best remedies for **nose-bleeds** with bright red blood. It is especially useful for those tired, anemic looking children or adolescents who typically faint from the sight of blood.

Ferrum phos. is also useful for the very *first stage* **of colds,** ear infections, sore throats, tracheitis and lung problems, where there are no symptoms except a fever (what we call a "low-grade **fever of unknown origin**"). It is often used as a convalescent remedy for children who remain **tired and sickly looking** after a viral infection.

Gelsemium sempervirens *(yellow jasmine)*

Gelsemium is characterized by the "D's": **drowsy, dopey, dizzy, dumb, disoriented** and **dull.** You can see right away why it is such a **classic flu** remedy. The person feels all of the above "as if a truck drove over me." He has **chills** going up and down the spine, he feels so **tired** that he thinks he cannot even lift his finger to take something and he even has aching upon moving his eyes. Yet he **can't fall asleep**. Curiously enough, in spite of the fever, he has absolutely **no thirst** and a **slow pulse**! Symptoms are made worse by motion, light, noise and stuffy rooms. There is **trembling** although the person is listless and has low stamina. The flu is accompanied by a headache. Gelsemium was the main remedy for the 1996-97 flu epidemic!

Besides being good for flu, Gelsemium is a great remedy for **"hearing bad news"**: the person reacts to hearing bad news (for example a doctor saying that your mammogram is positive and it might be cancer) as if she is paralyzed, she can't move, she just sits there, **trembling**.

It is also effective for fright with trembling after **earthquakes** and in case of **anticipation anxiety** (like Argentum nitricum). However, unlike with Argentum nitricum (where the anxiety can start weeks in advance), with Gelsemium the anticipation anxiety starts just before the event takes place; for example, you have a speaking engagement, everything seems to be all right until you have to start speaking, then you are overcome with fear and trembling.

Gelsemium is the #1 remedy for **fear of the dentist,** and I give it to my dog when he has to go to the vet. It is greatly indicated in **headaches**, especially ones preceded by an aura of blurred vision and improved when the person **passes great amounts of urine**. In the past, acute cases of polio were cured by Gelsemium.

Glonoin *(nitroglycerin)*

Since Glonoin is made from nitroglycerin—used to make dynamite—you can guess what it is used for:

a "bomb of a headache!" These are what Western medicine calls **"cluster" headaches**, with violent rushes of blood to the head, sensations of throbbing and expanding, not responding to any medication. Usually lasting for more than a day, a Glonoin headache is sheer agony for the person. Glonoin is also good for headaches **after sunstroke** or from too long exposure to the sun.

Hepar sulphuris *(a type of calcium sulphide)*

Hepar sulph., made from a chemical compound invented by Hahnemann, is still totally unknown in Western science. It is mostly used in homeopathy to stimulate the suppuration (pus formation) or **ripening of an abscess or boil**. It is indicated in any condition where there is inflammation with a tendency to suppuration. The person is apt to be very sensitive to pain and the slightest draft of air. There can be a **sensation "as if there is a splinter"** in the tissues (throat, anus, etc.). There is a great desire for **vinegar** and sour things.

Hepar sulph. is greatly indicated in **left-sided sore throats** which are relieved by drinking hot drinks. It is also effective for the typical **candida yeast discharge** (cottage cheese-like discharge); all discharges have a spoiled cheese smell. A final use is to remove an infected **splinter** which is too deeply lodged for tweezers; after a couple of doses of Hepar sulph. to ripen the infection, give Silica to expel the splinter. (If the splinter is not infected, you can just give Silica to push it out.)

Hydrastis canadensis *(goldenseal!)*

Hydrastis is very well-known and overused in tincture form in healthfood stores, where it is usually combined with echinacea and touted to boost the immune system. However, goldenseal in tincture (like echinacea or any other medicinal herb) should be used sparingly, only in acute colds or flus, and not on a continuous basis as advertised, or else it is bound to backfire and cause the same symptoms it tries to combat.

Hydrastis is a great **sinusitis** remedy, often following Pulsatilla in our prescriptions as it is effective for **thick, yellow, sticky mucus,** often associated with burning pains. It is also the greatest remedy for dyspepsia or **maldigestion** (along with Nux vomica), and for **gastritis** with dull pains in the stomach and a feeling of emptiness in the pit of the stomach (like Sulphur). In the past, homeopathic prescribers often used this remedy for cancers of the stomach, liver and colon.

Hypericum perforatum *(St. John's wort)*

Hypericum, or St. John's wort, has recently become recognized in the medical community as an antidepressant, touted as the natural alternative to Prozac. It is ironic that Hypericum as a homeopathic remedy has had those anti-depressive characteristics for 200 years (long before the medical society stumbled on it). However, in homeopathy it is certainly not the top remedy for depression! We have many other remedies which are even more effective in treating depression.

Hypericum is much more useful as a great **painkiller** in any trauma which involves **nerve endings**: **slipped discs** in sciatica, slipped discs in the neck, **crushed fingers** (when you slam the door inadvertently on your child's hand or a fingernail has been ripped off). Hypericum is for sharp, shooting nerve pains, so it can also be used in **toothaches** with such pains, or after an **insect or animal bite** (in fact it is the #1 remedy for dog bites). Having studied neurology, I wish neurolgists would give Hyper. routinely after **spinal taps** as it provides immediate relief for the dreaded headache which so often follows this procedure. In the past it was given successfully to avoid tetanus.

Ignatia amara *(St. Ignatius' bean)*

Even if homeopathy had only produced this remedy, it would be worth it! There are probably very few people on earth who will never need this remedy. Indeed it is indicated in **acute grief** events and emotional shocks, mainly related to relationships. Any broken heart situation should be remedied by Ignatia: the person has the **"3 S"** symptoms: **sitting, sighing, and sobbing**. She laments, "Why me, God, why is it happening to me?"

But don't try to console her, or she will turn on you in a rage. Then this crying can turn into hysterical, uncontrollable laughing. People who need Ignatia have very **changeable moods!** We can call it the "homeopathic Valium" as it is also used in any event where you get **upset**: bad news, disappointment (especially in relationships with friends, family, lovers, children, etc.), apprehension and jealousy.

Typical symptoms include a sensation **"as if there is a lump in the throat"** preventing the person from swallowing, yet they can swallow. The person may go to bed and be unable to fall asleep as she keeps on thinking about what has happened to her: it is called the **rehearsal** remedy as the person tries in vain to flee those painful memories. They dream all night about the same subject, dreams full of disappointment and unfulfilled expectations. Symptoms also tend to be worse **premenstrually and around 11 a.m.**

Ipecac (Ipecacuanha) *(a Brazilian shrub)*

Ipecac syrup is very well known in Western medicine to induce vomiting. Thus, following the prin-

107

ciple of "like cures like," it is used in homeopathy to relieve vomiting with strong nausea (just the thought of food gags the person). This could be the case during pregnancy (morning sickness), after over–medication or strong medications, to help AIDS patients with these complaints, for the typical summer flus which can lead to dehydration, or simply in indigestion.

A typical symptom for Ipecac is that vomiting does not relieve the nausea and that the person has a clean tongue (the opposite of what we would expect when the person has such severe gastrointestinal symptoms). The person is not thirsty.

Ipecac is indicated in acute asthma and migraine attacks, accompanied with nausea or menstrual cramps, as it is a major anti-spasmodic remedy. It is a great remedy for coughs, especially with gagging at the end (not surprisingly, considering its connection with vomiting).

Kali bichronicum *(potassium bichromate)*

Kali bich. is a remedy my patients get to know fast and very well: they see the miracles it works in cases of **congestion in the sinuses** and the face in general, with **postnasal drip** playing havoc with its victim. It can cut through the **thick, sticky yellow-green mucus** ("when it sticks, use Kali Bich.!") so often observed nowadays in our children who are great "mucus producers." They often gag on their mucus, especially at night where the viscous mucus gets stuck in the throat, making breathing increasingly difficult. The discharge during the day flows and then it stops, repeated in cycles.

My patients have often found that they need to use Kali bich. by the tablespoonful rather than the teaspoonful to loosen this particularly stubborn, sticky type of mucus.

Kali bich. can also be used for pain sharply localized on **small spots** (the person can put a finger on the painful spot). The pains start and stop suddenly, and they are worse from exposure to cold and from **drinking beer,** which stuffs up the nose immediately. Coughing (often around 2 or 3 a.m.) is followed by the difficult expectoration of that stringy mucus.

While the layperson mainly uses Kali bich. for colds, flus and sinusitis, there are many other acute indications, including thick green vaginal discharge and **headaches** above the eyeballs, even migraines preceded by visual disturbances.

Kali phosphoricum *(potassium phosphate)*

Kali phos. has a great action on the nervous system. Students and others suffering from depression and exhaustion after **prolonged intellectual work** can benefit from this remedy. The brain fatigue leads to loss of memory, **headaches in school children** (also relieved by Calc. phos.) and a feeling of physical as well as mental exhaustion. So it is great for ailments from overstudy, as well as for ailments from **night–watching** (like Cocculus), where the person has lost a lot of sleep while taking care of an ill family member or friend.

Ledum palustre *(wild rosemary)*

Ledum acts like a combination of Arnica and Hypericum. So often it will completely relieve traumas after the initial use of Arnica. I think about it especially for **black eyes** (the #1 remedy), and for bruises when they have turned violet-blue-black. It has an equally great effect on puncture wounds (which do not bleed long) caused by a sharp instrument The pains relieved by Ledum are improved by cold compresses and cold water in general.

Ledum is great for all kinds of **insect bites,** and I have often gotten great relief from this remedy during my travels when I was visited at night by uninvited **mosquitoes**. Think also about your beloved dogs and help them with **flea bites**: give them Ledum 200C in water, just as you would take it yourself, repeating it as needed.

It is unfortunate that hospitals have not discovered the magic of this remedy for **bedsores**. Nurses, often overwhelmed by work, don't always have the time to turn their bedridden patients on a regular basis, and often we see painful, awful-looking bed-sores on these poor victims.

Other uses of Ledum include acute **gout** attacks in the big toe, and **hangovers** after **whiskey** and other hard liquor. It should be routinely given *after* **vaccinations** (whether to your children or your animals) to counteract the bad effects of vaccinations (one dose of Ledum 200C is sufficient, three pellets dry, in the mouth).

Lycopodium clavatum *(club moss)*

Lycopodium is a great remedy for the liver and gastrointestinal tract. For example, it is a great remedy for **constipation**, typically occurring when you **travel**. When this constipation is accompanied by great **bloating below the navel** (you look five months pregnant after a meal!), even after a few mouthfuls of food with **fermentation** in intestines—especially after cabbage, beans and onions—and strong **cravings for sweets**, then Lycopodium will come to the rescue.

It's important to remember that all complaints relieved by Lycopodium are typically **worse from 4-8 p.m.** and better after midnight, better from hot food and drinks but worse from being in a warm room. Complaints are mainly **right-sided.** Lycopodium can also be indicated when complaints go from right to left, as in a sore throat. Sore throats relieved by drinking hot liquids are also likely to respond to Lycopodium. Another indication is a dry tickling cough at night. Acid indigestion, often leading to headaches, will also respond to Lycopodium.

The emotional picture of this remedy (for people who need it in chronic diseases) is one of very **low self-confidence**, especially for any new task or anything out of the ordinary routine. There is a great fear of failure and a child will constantly say, "I can't do this." Therefore, the child often keeps postponing his homework (further lowering his self-esteem) and struggles with his parents. The result is often a diagnosis of ADD (Attention Deficit Disorder). So Lycopodium is a great remedy for this type of ADD, as well as for dyslexia problems (your homeopathic physician should decide this!). The low self-confidence exhibited by people who need this remedy often stems from a **humiliation, fear, fright or betrayal** situation.

Magnesia phosphorica *(magnesium phosphate)*

Like any Magnesium compound, Mag. phos. will work great for cases of spasms and **cramps**. This is seen best in conditions like dysmenorrhea (**painful menses**) or in leg cramps (**charley horses**). The pains start and end **suddenly**, nerve-like pains which makes the person cry out loud, and **are relieved by**

bending over (doubling up) and by **heat**. Colicky babies have been helped by this remedy, as well as cramps in violin players (player's cramp), in sciatica and facial nerve pain. Keep in mind that it is mainly a **right-sided** remedy (Colocynth is a left-sided remedy with similar characteristics; see listing under Colocynth). Mag. phos. and Cuprum will resolve 90% of leg and foot cramps.

Mercurius vivus or solubilis *(mercury)*

Think of Mercury as the **human thermometer**: complaints change or aggravate with the slightest change of weather. People needing Merc. show their low resistance to temperature change by their difficulty adjusting to variations in temperature and their low resistance to colds and flus. They lack a normal defense mechanism and lose energy suddenly when suffering from colds.

The controversy about mercury in dental fillings has been around for some time, with several European countries forbidding mercury dental fillings. In the U.S. no such stand has been taken, but many people concerned with their poor health or compromised immune system have undergone the painful and expensive process of having their mercury fillings removed. Fortunately, from homeopathy we know that some people will benefit from this while others will not; and we know the symptoms of mercury toxicity (which are the same as the symptoms experienced in a proving of homeopathic Mercurius). Thus it is possible to predict in an individual case whether removing mercury fillings will improve overall health. These symptoms include:

- **Increased salivation** with intense thirst, especially at night; one would find saliva on the pillow in the morning. This symptom is so specific for Merc. that we can almost prescribe on this symptom alone.

- A tendency to **heavy sweating** especially at night; the increased perspiration does not relieve the complaints or make the person feel better. It can be looked at as a source of energy loss.

- Foul-smelling breath, **bleeding gums, a metallic taste** in the mouth, a mapped tongue (with patches of different colors), the imprint of the teeth along the side of the tongue, **trembling tongue** when the tongue is protruded.

- A tendency to **abscessed teeth** and sore throats with **enlarging of the lymph nodes,** and pus on the tonsils (the typical strep throat).

- **Canker sores** and herpes sores in the mouth.

As one can see, many Merc. symptoms are located in the mouth, making it the worst place in our bodies to introduce mercury in the form of dental fillings.

There are many uses for Mercurius. The most common include **sore throats** (whole throat) with **swollen glands** and constant inclination to swallow; **mumps** (although Jaborandi is the #1 remedy); and **ear infections** with green, yellowish thick discharge.

Whenever you are going to have mercury dental fillings removed, protect yourself by taking Merc. 200C or 30C (3 pellets dry) before the procedure as well as afterwards. This will minimize the danger from the mercury released during extraction; otherwise extreme fatigue and malaise are often seen after such an intervention.

Mezereum *(spurge olive)*

Mezereum is a great skin remedy. For our purposes, the main indication is for the brutal, lingering pains after the herpes-like lesions of shingles (herpes zoster) have disappeared. Not uncommonly, the person suffers more from these **postzonal neuralgias** (as we call them in medicine) than from the original shingles attack. There is violent burning and itching in the blister-like eruptions; the person scratches until they bleed, and then there is crust formation. Mezereum is also an excellent remedy for impetigo (although Ant-crud. is the first choice).

Nux vomica *(poison chestnut)*

Here's news for those of you who believe in curing a hangover with the proverbial raw egg in a pot of coffee. A **hangover from alcohol** (especially from beer) can be relieved as if by magic with a few pellets of Nux vomica.

Nux vomica is used in **gastric** conditions in general; it relieves the pains and bloating from overeating, especially from **fatty and rich foods** or too much **coffee**. It's the perfect remedy for the sedentary business person, plagued by constipation, gas and burping, and craving stimulants like coffee and alcohol. It will relieve indigestion with a feeling **"as if there is a weight in the stomach"** about one to two hours after eating. It will also relieve constipation with the typical **ineffective urging**: the person keeps trying to defecate, always feeling that there is more to come out. I have seen nothing better for the constipation of a newborn baby. People who have longterm **constipation after taking too many laxatives** can be helped by Nux vomica, although they should do so under the care of a homeopathic physician.

Nux vomica is also a major remedy for alcoholics, as well as for hayfever attacks with spasmodic sneezing in the morning upon awakening **(with the nose stopped up at night and runny in the day).**

Another great situation for Nux vomica is **insomnia** due to **stress at work**: the person takes his problems to bed and typically awakens at **3 a.m.**, tossing and turning, thinking about what he did yesterday and what he has to do tomorrow. Of course he feels unrefreshed and groggy ("as if he has a hangover") upon awakening. Only a cup of coffee seems to get him going, but this leads to a vicious cycle requiring more and more coffee.

Petroleum *(coal oil)*

Petroleum is mainly known as a skin remedy in eczema. It is also excellent for **seasickness** (like Tabacum). It works equally well against the acute blisters of herpes (like Rhus tox. and Nat. mur.). Another unusual use is in cases of **diarrhea from cabbage or sauerkraut**.

Phosphoricum acidum *(phosphoric acid)*

Phos. acid. is a great remedy for grief, especially in cases of **homesickness** (like Capsicum). The person feels extreme weakness and **indifference**, even to things he normally enjoys. He lies down with his face to the wall, unplugs the phone and does not want to communicate with anyone. The grief literally drains him and often evolves to depression. There is a **loss of memory** and spaciness, with drowsiness by day and insomnia at night. Phos. acid. is the most prominent remedy for **unrefreshed sleep**.

117

People who need Phos. acid. typically refuse to eat, except they crave sour things and fruits which cause a **painless diarrhea** which does not fatigue the person. They also crave sodas and carbonated drinks. (Not coincidentally, phosphoric acid is used to make the bubbles in cola drinks and other sodas.).

Phosphorus *(white phosphorus)*

More about this wonderful remedy is written in Part Five. It has numerous uses, including **bleeding disorders** (bright red blood, without a tendency to clot) nose bleeds, and bleeding after surgery or a tooth extraction, overly heavy menstrual cycles, post–partum bleeding, etc. In these situations it stops the bleeding rapidly. It should be taken before any surgical intervention, as close to surgery time as possible, and again afterwards if bleeding is a problem.

Phosphorus is used for many lung conditions (such as **viral pneumonia**) with a hard, racking, burning cough, worse from lying on the left side. It is also used for sore throats where the person cannot talk because of pain in the larynx.

If only people who have been **struck by lightning** knew about Phosphorus. This phenomenon is not as rare as one would suspect; support groups are everywhere for these unfortunate people who complain of fatigue and headaches after being struck by a bolt of lightning. Phosphorus would be the perfect remedy for this and for severe electric shocks.

Phosphorus is also used for many **hypoglycemic** conditions. And **Calc. phos. 6X** (a cell salt, calcium phosphate) is the greatest remedy for preventing and treating **osteoporosis** (3 pellets dry, in the mouth, daily). People who are constitutionally a Phosphorus type (described in Part Five) are especially susceptible to this condition.

Phytolacca decandra *(pokeweed)*

Phytolacca is a great remedy for glandular and cystic conditions. It is especially helpful in common cystic breast conditions as it has a great action on the mammary glands. It will help with very painful breast abscess and mastitis during breast feeding. If the breasts are painful and swollen before the menstrual cycle, Phytolacca will give quick relief.

Phytolacca also relieves right-sided sore throats with a dark-red appearance and swollen glands, pains radiating to the ear, worse from drinking warm drinks. When Phytolacca is needed, there is a sensation of stiffness and bruising all over the body (like Rhus tox. and Arnica). It is an excellent remedy for sciatica in which there is stiffness and pain which forces the person to move, but then the person does not feel better from the movement (as they would if they needed Rhus tox.).

119

Podophyllum *(May-apple)*

There is no remedy like Podophyllum for **children's diarrhea:** watery, large quantities preceded by rumbling in the abdomen, **relieved by lying on the stomach**. It also relieves summer diarrhea after eating **too much fruit** (like Phos. acid.). Like Chamomilla, it is a remedy for diarrhea after **teething**, worst in the early morning (4 a.m.), and worse after drinking milk.

Pulsatilla *(wind flower)*

The personality of Pulsatilla as a constitutional remedy type is further discussed in Part Five. A great characteristic of Pulsatilla—corresponding to its mental indecisiveness and emotional moodiness—is that the symptoms are never the same: they swing from one extreme to another, or there is **constant changeability**. The mucus expectoration may be first green, then yellow, then white, constantly changing. The symptoms are always **worse in a warm room and around 5 p.m.** or after sunset; they are **better in cool fresh air** and when the person is moving slowly. The person who needs Pulsatilla has **no thirst** even when they have a fever, the exact opposite of what you would expect.

Pulsatilla is often used for **sinusitis** with stuffiness hindering nose-breathing and with the production of yellow, white mucus. It's also used for

itching of the eyes at night in allergies. It is definitely the most widely used remedy for various **childhood diseases**: measles, mumps, German measles, and chickenpox. It can be used preventively as well as curatively: if there is an epidemic of one of these diseases in your neighborhood, protect your children with 3 pellets of Pulsatilla 200C, dry in the mouth, daily as long as they are being exposed.

Pulsatilla is also good for frostbite, and for diarrhea or headaches from eating icecream or fruit. It is one of the main remedies (along with Sepia and Ipecac) for morning sickness and vomiting during pregnancy. And it is definitely the #1 remedy for the **late onset of menses** in any young girl displaying the well-known Pulsatilla emotional state (easy weeping, neediness for consolation, shyness, moodiness and changeable behavior).

Ranunculus bulbosus *(buttercup)*

Ranunculus has a great action on the skin, especially for skin conditions that tend to form blisters or little vesicles like **Herpes zoster**. It is the #1 remedy for acute outbreaks of shingles, especially on the ribcage. The blisters often contain a liquid which gives them a bluish color. It helps greatly to relieve the acute, shooting pains, worse when touched, which are typical of shingles, a condition affecting many people under great stress. It also relieves the pain of the shingles around the eye (the ophthalmic variation of Herpes zoster).

Rhus toxicodendron *(poison ivy)*

As its name indicates, Rhus tox. is a good remedy for **poison ivy,** although Anacardium is the # 1 remedy for this painful, debilitating affliction. But the symptoms associated with Rhus tox. indicate many more uses for it. All symptoms responding to Rhus tox. are **better with heat** (such as a hot shower) and **continued movement;** they are made **worse by humidity** (thus it is called the human barometer as the person can predict the weather better than any forecaster), worse when **beginning to move** (the first steps), and **worse from resting.** The person needing Rhus tox. feels better once he has overcome the initial stiffness and the movement is underway (the "rusty gate" syndrome). The sensation of **stiffness** is especially in the **joints** (in Arnica it is in the muscles).

Rhus tox. is also used acutely to relieve **herpes** lesions (cold sores, genital herpes) and also **sciatica** with stiffness and tearing pains, which feel better when the person is moving around and worse when he is resting. Like Ant. tart. and Pulsatilla, Rhus tox. is a good remedy for chickenpox. It is the best remedy for any **sprain or strain affecting ligaments** anywhere in the body. Together with Arnica (for sore muscles), it will bring great relief to athletes who have overexerted themselves.

Rumex crispus *(yellow dock)*

Made from a plant used in herbal medicine, Rumex is very useful for **coughs**, especially those that get **worse when uncovering** (like undressing); it is a constant dry cough worse when breathing in cold air (like a Phosphorus cough). The cough is relieved when the person covers his mouth with his hand. It is also used for **skin** conditions in which **itching** starts when undressing at night. Sometimes it helps to expectorate thick stubborn mucus in the chest.

Ruta graveolens *(rue, bitterwort)*

Ruta combines characteristics of Arnica and Rhus tox. It is mainly indicated when there is a deeper trauma to the soft tissues so that the **periosteum** (the membrane surrounding the bone) has been affected. A classic example of this is its great effectiveness for **tennis elbow** (like Bellis perennis), where the trauma is close to the bone. There will be a feeling of stiffness as in conditions relieved by Rhus tox., and a bruised feeling as in Arnica conditions. Moving around makes the pains worse.

Ruta has a great action on the **knee** and is therefore indicated in any trauma to the knee. It is the #1 remedy for injuries to the **Achilles tendon**. When one has read too much or sat in front of the computer too much, a few pellets of Ruta will relieve the **eye strain**.

Sambucus nigra *(black elder)*

Sambucus is a great whooping cough and acute asthma remedy, in which the person wakes up at night from the cough with an intense feeling of suffocating and being unable to exhale. These attacks tend to be worst at 2 or 3 a.m. The person cannot lie down but instead feels better from sitting up or needs to get out of bed and walk around. It is interesting to know that the juice of black elder is used to lose weight.

Sanguinaria canadensis *(bloodroot)*

Sanguinaria is a great remedy for **right-sided headaches** with throbbing pains, beginning in the back of the head and radiating until they end above the right eye. These headaches have a **periodicity**; in this case they occur **every seven days** or every other day. It also relieves **right-sided frozen shoulder.**

Sepia *(ink of the cuttlefish or giant squid)*

What a great remedy to **restore the physical and emotional powers** to a woman who is **worn out** from too many pregnancies, abortions or miscarriages, too much and too early responsibility (like a 12-year-old girl taking over the role of her absent mother), or simply too much work at home: children, husband, and career which she has seemingly juggled with great endurance until she finally has had it. She is over-whelmed by work and reponsibilities.

Then there is only one way out: escaping to a silent place, by herself, with great indifference to anyone as she feels she cannot entertain anyone. Away from the daily chores! Away from the ever-demanding daily routine of feeding her kids, bring-ing them to soccer practice—and then there is the "big boy" asking for sex to which she has great aversion. The woman in a Sepia state cannot bear it. She wants to run away, as far as possible. When-ever you recognize the above situation, whenever you are "dead" emotionally and physically, you should run—to your homeopathic physician, who will help you before you resort to smacking your children.

As for our acute uses, Sepia relieves morning sickness. It is definitely the #1 remedy for **preg-nancy vomiting** and for **prolapse of the organs** (bladder, uterus). The #1 remedy for **leucorrhea** (vaginal discharge, "the whites") in little girls, Sepia also relieves **itching of the vagina** with great **dryness** commonly seen in menopause. Sepia is a great remedy for menopause in general, especially when hot flushes and hair loss are present.

As you can see, most of the uses for Sepia are chronic in nature and require assistance from your homeopathic physician, but I could not omit this important remedy. Any working woman has been in this situation at some point. For a more complete description, see the section on Sepia in Part Five.

Silicea *(silicon dioxide, quartz crystal)*

Silicea should be a must after every **DPT vaccination** as it can protect against the bad effects of vaccinations in general and especially DPT (give 200C, three pellets dry, in the mouth, *after* the vaccination). It has a remarkable power to push **splinters** to the surface and has been called the "homeopathic surgical knife." Silicea is also used for **boils** to help them ripen or come to a head (what we call stimulating suppuration), and also in styes and abscesses. It will help close **fistulas** (although this should be under the care of your physician).

Silicea is a great remedy for many different nail conditions, such as white spots, ingrown toenails, and brittle nails. It also helps relieve **foot sweat** (and by the way, never use a commercial preparation to suppress sweat on the feet or anywhere else on the body, because blocking the body's natural outlet for any discharge can cause much worse health problems later on).

Spigelia marilandica *(pinkroot)*

Spigelia is a great remedy for **left-sided headaches**

when the headache starts in the neck and then radiates to the front of the head, finally stopping above the left eye (compare Sanguinaria for headaches above the right eye and Silicea for headaches above both eyes). Spigelia is also one of the best remedies for a very painful condition called **trigeminal neuralgia** on the left side of the face (although this too should be under the care of a professional).

Spongia tosta *(toasted sea sponge)*

Spongia is very well-known as a cough remedy for the **dry, hacking, croupy,** barking cough, day *and* night, exhausting the person. This cough tends to be worst at midnight (like Aconite) and **better when the person drinks hot liquids**. It is usually called for when the cough starts after being exposed to dry cold winds (again, like Aconite). It is one of the great croup remedies, along with Hepar sulph and Aconite.

Stannum metallicum *(the metal tin)*

Stannum is well-known for its effects in lung conditions accompanied by great weakness, expressed by a very weak voice and shortness of breath with the slightest effort, so that the person can hardly talk because of weakness. The person is also likely to cough up a great deal of greyish or yellow mucus, or mucus that looks like the white of an uncooked egg. The symptoms get worse from any exertion, from ascending stairs, at night, and upon exposure to cold.

127

Staphysagria *(stavesacre, larkspur)*

While this remedy is very useful in many physical illnesses, I want to direct your attention first to its great healing power in what we can call ***indignation/ humiliation situations*** of physical, emotional, mental, sexual and/or verbal abuse. The repetition of these events creates a climate in which the woman is not able to stand up to her abuser (suppressed anger). Anyone caught in a bad abusive relationship or marriage should be helped by this remedy (but only with the guidance of your homeopathic physician).

Staphysagria should be given immediately to any **rape** victim (after Arnica for the physical bruises) to heal the devastating emotional effects. It is also of great effect in **"honeymoon cystitis,"** so-called for its prevalence after increased sexual intercourse (because a woman's body can experience sex as an invasion or trauma, even when it is desired emotionally). Likewise if you have to undergo a **cystoscopy** (bladder examination) or **catheterization**, you should take Staphysagria as long as the catheter is in place. It will avoid pains and infections in the urethra. In fact it should be used preventively *before* these operations (200C, 3 pellets dry in the mouth) to prevent pain and infection.

Staphysagria is the #1 remedy for **styes**, for which it has a quick curing effect. I have used it preventively for **mosquito bites** (take a 30C dry every morning when you are in mosquito country).

Sulphur *(the mineral sulphur)*

Sulphur is one of our top remedies for **rashes, eczemas** and other skin conditions. For example, Sulphur is a must for a baby born with eczema after its mother took prescription medications during pregnancy. Sulphur will clear the drugs out of the baby's system, clear up the rash and relieve the unbearable **itching and burning.**

Sulphur is a much safer way to treat skin conditions than cortisone creams, zinc ointments, or other topical treatments which only drive the condition deeper inside the body. Many times we homeopaths see children suffering from asthma or convulsions as a direct result of skin conditions suppressed with cortisone. Western medicine still does not recognize such devastating longterm effects, a heavy price to pay for temporary relief of surface symptoms.

Other uses for Sulphur include hot flashes in menopause; recurrent styes (although Staph. is the #1 remedy); and **reducing cravings for alcohol** and detoxifying the liver in alcoholics, along with Nux vomica. It can also be used with Nux vomica to shrink hemorrhoids, thereby avoiding surgery. (In this case take Nux vomica 6C in the morning and Sulphur 6C in the evening; first check with your homeopathic physician).

Symptoms associated with Sulphur are always

worse during the **night,** in the **warmth of the bed,** and while taking a **hot shower** or bath. The itching and burning becomes so intolerable that the person scratches until he bleeds.

For a portrait of the mental and emotional characteristics of this remedy, please see Part Five.

Symphytum officinale *(comfrey)*

Symphytum is the great remedy to accelerate **healing of fractures** *after* the bone has been set. (In fact it is so effective that you should make sure the broken bone is aligned correctly before starting the remedy.) Symphytum is also used for **trauma to the eye** due to the blow of a fist while the surrounding soft parts remain intact (i.e. when the bones of the eye are fractured; for a black eye from soft tissue damage, use Ledum).

Tabacum *(tobacco)*

This is the only way we should take tobacco: in homeopathic doses! Nothing works better for **seasickness** than this remedy. And guaranteed, no drowsiness. Take a dose one hour before you go on the boat (200C, 3 pellets dry, in the mouth) and repeat if needed.

Urtica urens *(stinging nettle)*

Urtica urens is a remedy that made Dr. Compton

Burnett famous a hundred years ago. With his "secret potion" this English homeopath cured so many cases of gout that he was known all over Europe as "Dr. Gout." After his death, his family divulged the contents of his secret formula—consisting primarily of this one simple homeopathic remedy!

Even today, Urtica urens is capable of helping to ward off a severe acute attack of **gout.** Another great indication is **urticaria (hives),** particularly after eating **seafood** or cheese. The symptoms are **stinging,** burning and severe itching, all of which are quickly alleviated by Urtica urens. It is also useful for **first degree burns,** for **stings from jellyfish** and bees, and for rashes caused by the stinging nettle plant itself.

Veratrum album *(white hellebore)*

Veratrum album was one of the three great remedies Hahnemann successfully used two hundred years ago to eradicate **cholera** epidemics (the others were Camphor and Cuprum). And of course it can still cure cholera even today.

For the layperson, Veratrum is a great remedy for **summer diarrheas** with vomiting, extreme fatigue, and **cold sweat,** especially on the forehead; the hands can also be icy cold. The person is **very thirsty** and desires cold drinks, often with **ice cubes.** He also desires **salty foods** and sour foods (like pickles and lemons). This type of diarrhea can lead to dehydration and collapse if left untreated.

Veratrum is useful in general for **hypovolemic shock** (shock resulting from loss of fluids, whether from vomiting, diarrhea, etc.). You might confuse some of the symptoms of Veratrum with Arsenicum, but the person who needs Arsenicum is restless and anxious, while the person needing Veratrum is quiet.

Zincum metallicum *(metal zinc)*

Zincum is the best remedy for a **hangover** after drinking excessive amounts of **wine,** or for someone who is affected by even small amounts of wine. It has also greatly helped in **"restless leg syndrome"** which prevents the person from sleeping.

PART FIVE

Brief Portraits of Some Well-Known Remedies

- ❖ *Sulphur*

- ❖ *Phosphorus*

- ❖ *Calcarea carbonica*

- ❖ *Pulsatilla*

- ❖ *Natrum muriaticum*

- ❖ *Sepia*

Many of the homeopathic remedies have such striking mental and emotional symptoms associated with them that they can be recognized as personality types. A few of the most common remedy types are presented here. If you can recognize your friends and family members in these portraits, not only will you gain a deeper understanding of their moods and behavior, but you will also know what remedies they are most likely to need when they fall ill.

The Sulphur Personality: A General at Work

As a child, the Sulphur person already stands out. You can see right away that he will be a leader rather than a follower. Even as young as two years old, the child shows his independence by wanting to run away from his mother. These are the toddlers whose mothers have to put them on a little leash when they go out. The Sulphur child is curious and explorative. As he grows up, other children tend to look up at him, as he commands attention through his strong personality. Other children like him because he has charisma and is fair in organizing games, where even the underdog is allowed to participate.

The Sulphur's disdain for external appearances shows up at young age. His hair flies all over the place, his shirt hangs out of his pants and he falls over his untied shoes. You never have to guess

Note: Sulphur is predominantly a male remedy, although this does not exclude the existence of female Sulphurs. But mostly the reader will recognize a male figure in this portrait.

To know more about the homeopathic personality types, please see my book *What About Men* or Catherine Coulter's *Portraits of Homeopathic Medicines,* one of the sources for these portraits (another being my observation of thousands of patients in my practice).

what he has eaten the previous night—the spaghetti spots testify to his ability to eat too much, too fast. He especially craves stimulating food like Chinese food, fried and fatty foods, and his all-time favorite, pizza. He is usually very intelligent, but that does not always work in his favor. He can be bored stiff when the teacher has to repeat himself for the slower children in his class. Often he "checks out" and starts daydreaming.

The Sulphur child is interested in factual things: he reads biographies, books about wars or the *Guinness Book of Records,* and is not at all interested in novels. This tendency persists throughout a Sulphur's life. Not uncommonly, a Sulphur boy will correct his teacher, to the amazement of the adult who cannot understand how this "lazy" boy knows these facts.

Puberty comes as a shock to many teenagers but especially to the Sulphur adolescent. He is very prone to skin conditions like disfiguring acne. Whereas before he did not care much about how he looked, now he sees his problem skin as an obstacle to his growing popularity among the girls. He will only agree to see a homeopath to get rid of these "zits"; he is not interested in improving anything else about himself.

As a teenager he still makes a mess of his room, and cleaning it up consists of sweeping his "stuff" into a cupboard. Waking up in the morning and getting ready to go to that boring school is as much of an ordeal as having all his teeth pulled out. He is grumpy, "not hungry" and prefers not to talk to anyone before ten a.m. But he always needs some money for snacking on the "nutritious" food from the school canteen. His popularity at school soars as he gets older, and he is often elected class president by his admiring fans.

Even at a young age the Sulphur recognizes the value of things. Pity the child who dares to enter into an exchange of collectibles with him. The Sulphur always comes out on top, although the other party never suspects this, the way he talks up the deal.

Of course, as a dynamo of energy he is a hot-blooded person. The Sulphur boy defines a sweater as something his mother pushes on him because *she* is cold. At night he usually throws off the blankets or at the very least, he sticks his feet out from under the covers. He considers taking showers a waste of water, and standing or sitting still is pure torture. Everything has to be fast, stimulating and exciting: music, computer games, movies, books, sports, etc.

The adult Sulphur will not change much. He just covers it up more to reap the full benefit of his behavior. He is still the man of action, the achiever and fierce competitor who can move mountains. He has just one great weakness: he can be pretty insensitive to his spouse because he is still very factual. This does not leave much room for sentiments. For example, he might keep an album with pictures of women he dated before he married his present wife, not realizing that this could appear insensitive.

If feelings come in the way of his plans, the Sulphur's motto is: "On we go!" He does not look back, holds no grudges, and easily moves on professionally and in his relationships. But he won't tolerate laziness either and will only respect people who work at least as hard as he does. When you first meet him, you might think that he is a jerk, intolerant of others when they do not reach their potential by *his* standards. He says that he has no sympathy for his "freeloading employees." Of course there is no place for tears or showing emotions. "That's for sissies," he says; a man should never cry, at least not in front of other people.

Mr. Sulphur usually has a physical appearance resembling a nervous race horse. He is lean and mean, although he can easily change to the opposite picture when he is burned out. At that point his cynicism takes over and he becomes the well-known philosopher: politics stink, newspapers lie, people are stupid, etc. It looks as though the only intelligent person is a Sulphur person, at least according to him; everyone else is a degree lower.

Sulphurs love being the center of the conversation, and they usually are, with their knowledge of facts. A Sulphur doesn't hesitate to jump, un-solicited, into his neighbor's conversation to give his view on the affair. He will not easily back off either. He can become quite quarrelsome and erupt like a volcano. Just remember one thing: these Sulphur outbursts are like real volcanic eruptions, rare and short-lived.

Mr. Sulphur loves a deal and would not hesitate to drive an extra five miles because the gasoline is two cents cheaper. And shopping at Marshall's or other discount stores is a must! He can be manic-depressive in the winter because the boredom of the winter plagues him. He thrives out-of-doors in the spring and summer. He never misses a day of work, which reflects his great energy and resilience. He appreciates a quick mind, wit and humor, something he is not devoid of himself.

And for a Sulphur, taking care of the family financially is his greatest achievement and concern. He is the one who should have been born a cave man so he could have "whacked the saber-toothed tiger on the head and brought him home for his wife to cook." He has a phenomenal memory, usu-ally photographic, which contrasts so much with the fact that he can't remember names, even of good friends. A Sulphur would reason that he never wants to become that personal, because it is a form of weakness.

A Sulphur's mind is always "preoccupied with higher things," so he is indifferent to what or when he eats. Don't ever expect him to pick up after himself. His desk is invariably covered with innumerable rings from cups and glasses. Dirty dishes pile up, as well as stacks of old newspapers, empty bottles, grocery bags, etc. representing his collector's mentality and his strange view of his possessions: if it's his, it's beautiful. So don't throw away an old pair of shoes or a ragged T-shirt, as these are his most prized possessions. He has almost no fears, except a fear of heights, where he feels that he is being drawn to the ground below if he risks looking downward.

A Sulphur is rarely depressed or discouraged. His outspokenness can cause many to dislike him. His utter conviction that he is right and everyone else wrong can easily make him enemies. The fact that he *is* frequently right does not ease matters. His ambition is fame, whatever it means and whatever it is worth. He is very tolerant about a person's sexual preference and will never pass judgment. As for himself, all the evidence shows that he is aggressively heterosexual.

All in all, a well-balanced Sulphur is witty, intelligent, hard-working, non-judgmental, a defender of the underdog and the general of the troops, not afraid to make decisions and change plans on the spur of the moment. If you have a Sulphur at home, you are in for the ride of your life, full of excitement and unexpected events. Enjoy!

A Sulphur person is likely to need these acute remedies:
Sulphurs are apt to get skin conditions like eczema, diaper rash and other rashes, for which **Sulphur** is an excellent acute remedy, as is **Graphites.**

Sulphurs are also prone to the ambitious, competitive, hardworking lifestyle—often associated with overindulgence in alcohol and other addictive and stimulating substances—which characterize a Nux vomica state. **Nux vomica** is an excellent remedy for the indigestion and hangovers which are likely to occur.

Sulphurs are also likely to have a sensitive digestive system and to suffer from gastrointestinal disturbances. **Lycopodium** is apt to be a good remedy for their gas, bloating and GI distress.

Finally, here is a tip which is useful for anyone who has had an Aconite cold (see Aconite in the *Guide to the Remedies)* which does not resolve completely. Take a dose of **Sulphur** 200C (3 pellets dry, in the mouth) and the fatigue, cough or other remnant will disappear. (Aconite is an acute remedy associated with Sulphur, which means that Sulphur people are more likely than others to get an **Aconite** cold.)

Phosphorus, the Sensitive and Excitable One

Attracting as much attention as the Sulphur, the luminescent Phosphorus personality is often his favorite companion. Rather than the charisma of the Sulphur, it is the external beauty and the liveliness of the Phosphorus person that makes heads turn. Even as a child, Phosphoruses attract attention with their big eyes, their long slender bodies and their eternal smile. Couple that with their uncanny ability for great communication and you have a winner. They love talking and have a great appreciation for friends, acquaintances and family, whom they support throughout any ordeal.

Empathy is second nature to a Phosphorus. It can be detrimental to her, though, as a Phosphorus is too sensitive and lacks boundaries. It is as though everything in her environment gets absorbed; she is like a psychogenic sponge "feeling yours and anyone else's pain." That leaves such a sensitive person on the verge of collapse, especially since a Phosphorus does not have the greatest physical and mental stamina in the first place.

Phosphoruses are not competitive in sports (although we can find some good runners among them), and too much studying leads to headaches and indifference. It is not that they lack intelligence. Like Sulphurs, Phosphoruses have a great memory, but they lack stamina. Therefore they are called great beginners and bad finishers. There is nothing better to revive a Phosphorus than a 30 minute nap; she feels reborn.

It is not only their lack of energy that contributes to their inability to finish, but also their sense of dissatisfaction and desire for change and excitement. They grow bored with the same things and that can extend to their life partner, from whom they demand continuous attention. Because of their beauty, they have no difficulty in finding other interested people. Sad to say, many Phosphorus people marry more than once because they grow tired of their present relationship.

We can easily see that a Phosphorus person belongs to the Heart-Fire-Joy element in the Five Elements of Traditional Chinese Medicine. They live for the present, spending money easily for beautiful clothes and expensive gadgets for their home, which they feel they should redecorate every six months (corresponding to their eternal restlessness). One item is never missing from the home of a Phosphorus: a mirror, or should we say many mirrors. They can't pass one without checking their hairdo, although they will claim that mirrors and self-portraits are just a way of enhancing the beauty of their house.

Beauty is very important to them. So don't insult a Phosphorus by asking her age; you won't get an answer. Although they always look at least ten years younger than they are, they have a fear of growing old and never dress the part. As one Phosphorus actress of 55 years old told me, "I can't play the role of a woman in her late twenties, but a thirty-year-old one, I can definitely play."

Invariably a Phosphorus will be inclined to dance, paint, sing, anything that creates beauty. From a young age they make their history lessons at school into an imaginary drama, with themselves at center stage, and they have a hard time with a too-structured teaching environment which does not allow for the spontaneity of a Phosphorus.

The sensitivity and active imagination of a Phosphorus leads to many anxieties and fears: fear of being alone, in the dark, ghosts, lightning, thunder, spiders, the future, death and incurable disease. They are fascinated by the subtle and vibrational spheres: meditation, crystals, channeling, or energy healing. They are the most spiritual and intuitive of the types. So a Phosphorus will be the first one to consult a medium or a fortune-teller. Nothing is more interesting than Nostradamus' predictions, and they won't hesitate to rearrange their lives around these fortunetellers. But they can easily be distracted from such gloomy predictions by plans for a party or a trip around the world.

Their physical sensitivity is a source of suffering for a Phosphorus. Perfumes, gasoline fumes, smoke, and even a great sensitivity to changes in the barometer, will aggravate existing symptoms or bring on headaches, fatigue and forgetfulness. If things get worse, they are the unfortunate souls who become allergic to the world and start reacting to everything: they can become prisoners in their own home, where everything has to be stripped bare and free of synthetics. You can imagine what that means for the sociable, adventure-traveling Phosphorus: it feels like a death sentence.

Otherwise a Phosphorus comes into this world with great assets: their beauty, intelligence, sparkle, sympathy, sensitivity, intuition, spirituality, romanticism and a great aesthetic sense.

A Phosphorus person is likely to need these acute remedies:
Phosphorus, not coincidentally, is the #1 remedy for many of the health concerns of a Phosphorus: a cough, for example (Phosphoruses are notoriously weak in the lung area) and easy bleeding (Phos–phoruses are the most likely to get nose bleeds, to bruise easily, and to have heavy menstrual periods with bright red blood, in all of which conditions the bleeding can be stanched by Phosphorus).

Phosphorus is also the best remedy for two other conditions which the sensitive Phosphorus person is most susceptible to: the bad effects of anesthesia and/or difficulty coming out of anesthesia; and a hypersensitivity to environmental chemicals, fumes, perfumes, etc.

Emotionally sensitive as they are, Phosphoruses are also the most likely to get into a **Nat. mur.** state (see the following portrait of Nat. mur.), which could possibly be avoided by taking **Ignatia** acutely.

The Calcarea Carbonicum: Down to Earth, and Not a Bad Bone in His Body

Many children in the U.S. are born this type: indeed, about 50% of them start out this way. And it is reflective of the steadiness and stubbornness of a Calc. carb. that many of them remain the same throughout their life. At birth they are grandmothers' favorites: big babies, with chubby cheeks inviting pinches and (in the grandmother's eye) radiating health and happiness.

Unfortunately, "fat and flabby" can remain a constant symptom, as they struggle with their weight for the rest of their life. But they are cute babies indeed, easily smiling and always having a great appetite (a breast is a pacifier for this baby and they make snacking an art form).

As part of their obstinacy, they have constipation from the beginning of their young life. They can go for days without a bowel movement, and that *without* any sign of discomfort. But watch out when they go! The bowel movements are voluminous and big, no one can believe that all this comes from such a little guy; not infrequently the mother has to break up the stool with a plunger so that it can be flushed down the toilet.

There is no other type as attached to their home as a Calc. carb. They are not interested in summer camp, especially if it is not right around the corner. I had knew a mother who kept making that mistake. Every summer, her little boy managed to misbehave so much at camp that he was sent home for the rest of the summer, where he then behaved perfectly in the company of a baby-sitter.

As you can see, the Calc. carb. is nice but stubborn. Moving away from a home is a catastrophe. Even if the new house is nicer and bigger, he will always miss that old house, the old neighborhood and his friends. In my practice I have often seen Calc. carb. suffer from a serious disease since moving away from his childhood home.

You have to think of a Calc. carb. person as an oyster (and indeed the remedy is made from the middle layer of the oyster shell): he has a hard shell (his stubbornness), but on the inside is this weak creature (the soft, flabby Calc. carb. person) and often you find a pearl of polished and delicate beauty—his compassionate, sensitive nature. He is horrified when he sees upsetting stories on TV. Often a Calc. carb. person does not read newspapers or turn on the TV for fear of seeing all the cruel things of this world—wars, famines and suffering. It really reflects the Calc. carb.'s great fear of physical harm and pain.

That's why the Calc. carb. child of three or four years old asks those questions about God and "What happens when I die?" Tell him some angels are waiting for him, who are going to play with him, and that there is going to be plenty of food (a major concern for a Calc. carb.!). He will be perfectly content as long as there is no suffering.

Just like a Phosphorus, a Calc. carb. can be very spiritual and giving, always ready to console people, to listen to their complaints, and then, alas, getting overwhelmed by it.

A Calc. carb. stands for the "F's": **fat, flabby, fair, faint, and fearful.** We have already discussed the lack of tone in this person ("there is little bounce to the ounce") and hence he is not readily interested in competitive sports, especially contact sports. He is exhausted from any physical effort, especially going upstairs. This includes sexual intercourse. In his thoughts he can be hypersexed, but in reality the act exhausts him as quickly as any other exercise.

Of the other F's, **faint** stands for the easy fainting this person goes through. As for **fearful**, nobody has more fears than a Calc. carb. I have already mentioned his fear of physical suffering, but this big, stout person is also fearful of mice, of the future, of death (there might be suffering), of disease (there is definitely suffering), of being alone (especially being away from home and mom), of poverty (no more food and no more safe home), of the dark (especially at night, when they always need a little light; Calc. carb. is a great remedy for the nightmares of children), and fear of changes (he likes routine, old friends, the same barber, the same doctor, etc.).

One sure thing is that a Calc. carb.'s appetite will never fail. He is a glutton and not very choosy about his foods, which can be plain and bland. Of course he never says no to ice cream or pizza, two of his more beloved foods. His wish list also includes boiled eggs and milk (which he tolerates poorly). He generally does not like meat (except for the occasional hamburger), but of course he would not say no to it if there is no other food. Fasting is definitely not in his vocabulary!

A Calc. carb. has a great sense of humor and likes teasing, which he does with an uncanny ability. But he is very sensitive to being teased himself. He can take quite a bit but he has his limits. Often the butt of the jokes at school, he can tolerate it for quite some time. But suddenly he will surprise everyone with a violent outburst—even to the point of killing someone. I have read about some of these unfortunate incidents in the newspapers. It is always incomprehensible to everyone involved that such a soft, mild, gentle child could suddenly kill someone (but no surprise if you know homeopathy!).

The Calc. carb. often shows his slowness early in life (late teething, late closing of the fontanels, late walking, late talking). At school the teacher can have the impression that he is not really intelligent as he will never volunteer to answer questions like the Sulphur (because he knows the answer) or the Phosphorus (anything to be loquacious and in the limelight). He sits in the background, but many times he will surprise peers and teachers alike by understanding everything and coming up with very logical answers. His logic is down-to-earth.

I had a four-year-old patient who heard his mother saying that his pediatrician had moved. The next time he felt sick, he did not say anything. When the mother finally noticed his fever, she scolded him and asked him, "Why didn't you tell me?" The little fellow had a very logical answer: "My doctor moved, so there is no sense in complaining. He does not live in that office where I used to go."

A Calc. carb. never wants to get pressured into answering things, at school or at home. Even when I asked a little six-year-old Calc. carb., "Who is your best friend?" he answered, "I have to mull this over." (Quite the contrast to the Phosphorus girl who tells me she has fifty friends and can name them all; or the Sulphur boy who would look at me with disdain for asking such a stupid question, thinking "Doesn't he know, I am a Sulphur, so people admire me, and of course everyone *wants* to be my friend.")

Usually though, a Calc. carb. will tell me he has one very special friend who he prefers to spend his time with. But he never has any problems playing by himself, lining up his little cars against the wall or playing war with all his little characters, in quite an animated way for a Calc. carb. But you have to understand that he is in his own room in his own home, which he feels is his castle.

It is amazing that we see many of these characteristics maintained in the Calc. carb. adult. The Calc. carb. father lives for his family and friends. He loves to play cards and watch football while eating pizza. He adores his wife (who is often a Phosphorus trying to put some spice in his life). The Calc. carb. mother is pleased with staying at home, tending the garden, and driving the children to their various activities. She is the "mother on the block" for everyone who needs a sympathetic ear.

Calc. carbs. might appear naive, slow, and earthbound, but they have an unsurpassed inner beauty in the love they have for people and the earth. There are very stable people, contributing very much to happiness in this world.

A Calc. carb. person is likely to need these acute remedies: A Calc. carb. child is susceptible to recurring ear infections, especially those of a **Belladonna** type. When sick or under stress, he is also likely to become more clingy to his mother and demanding of attention, typical of conditions responding well to **Pulsatilla**.

One of Calc. carb.'s weak points is weak ligaments

and especially a weak back, which he is likely to strain by overlifting, a condition which responds well to **Rhus tox.** (the #1 remedy for lumbago).

And of course **Calc. carb.** will also be a good acute remedy for such common Calc. carb. problems as constipation and the ill effects of overwork, overworry and overlifting.

Pulsatilla:
Neediness for Attention

Have you ever seen a windflower in your garden? I remember seeing one in the yard of one of my students. It was a calm, windless day. Nothing moved except the little windflower: it was swaying from one side to another, like a pendulum. Keep that image in your mind and you will know what a Pulsatilla person stands for. Indeed, changeability is Pulsatilla's great characteristic.

You can also call it irresolution: Pulsatilla can't make up her mind, whether choosing from a menu (more than one waiter has thought about committing hara-kiri because that sweet little Pulsatilla keeps on changing her main course) or when confronted with the 31 different flavors at a Baskin Robbins ice cream store. When a Pulsatilla buys some apples, she has to handle thirty of them before choosing the two she needs.

Note: I have referred mainly to *she* in talking about Phosphorus, Pulsatilla, Nat. mur. and Sepia, and mainly to *he* in discussing Sulphur, based on the predominance of the gender for each type. But this does not exclude the opposite sex from being any of these types. A Calc. carb. is equally likely to be male or female. We rarely see adult men who are Pulsatillas, but little boys who cling to their mothers can be.

And talk about Dr. Jekyll and Mr. Hyde—there is no better example than Pulsatilla. She has the uncanny ability to switch from one mood to the complete opposite within five minutes. Tears always seem to be present when needed for sympathy or attention, but the rainbow of smile and laughter always follows the rain.

It is hard to be angry at a little Pulsatilla child. She is sweet, always ready to help mummy in the kitchen, and constantly asking for approval from her mother. This is easily seen on a visit to the doctor. Ask her a question directly, and she will turn her head to mummy to make sure she gives the right answer. Or she may say, "You tell the doctor, mummy."

There is a sweetness and shyness about them, but don't be fooled. They have figured out at a very young age that you catch more flies with sugar than vinegar. Looking pretty, with such sweet behavior, dressed in their little dresses and sailor costumes, they can put a spell on you when you meet them. Hugs and kisses are demanded and given in equal amounts: who could ever say no to such a little princess?

Behind this smoke screen, though, there is a great hidden motive. They want constant attention; in fact there is no amount of love sufficient to fill the bottomless pit. Pulsatillas constantly demand proof of love. Comes the first day of school, they are a terror. They break their mother's heart with their piercing screams as they absolutely refuse to let go of mummy's hand, and the tortured mother is haunted by the screams of her sweet little princess as she leaves the school building.

For a Pulsatilla, this is sheer abandonment. "You don't love me anymore," they say. But once they adjust to the class, and especially if the teacher is gentle and pays attention to them, they love school. They become the teacher's pet, always ready to help. To the dismay of the Sulphurs and Phos–phoruses, they are the ones reminding the teacher that she forgot to give homework.

Imagine how upset a Pulsatilla is when a younger sibling is born. This is the greatest threat to their source of love: mom. All of a sudden their mother must pay attention to a little creature and Pulsatilla feels so abandoned. She refuses to visit mom in the hospital and does not want to kiss the new baby. If she can, she will pinch or hit the baby when no one is looking, or simply smack the door in the face of a younger sibling when he toddles innocently into the room. And of course, Pulsatilla will deny all of this.

If that does not work, there is the ultimate revenge. If mummy pays attention to a baby, she will resort to baby behavior. All of a sudden she wets her bed again, after being potty trained for the last three years. All of a sudden she loses her ability to dress herself. "Mummy, you help me put on this dress." No other child sucks on their thumb longer than a Pulsatilla. And if the baby's diaper gets changed, she wants something to be done for her too. This jealous behavior is always towards the younger sibling, not the older one.

When a Pulsatilla gets angry at mummy and storms into her room, she makes sure not to lock that door. She expects that mom is going to run after her, to take her into her arms and profess her deep love for her. Attention, attention—that's all she wants. When mom and dad are involved in a conversation, she keeps interrupting because she feels so excluded, and therefore abandoned. It is as if all the energy of a Pulsatilla is aimed at conquering love and attention.

Not all Pulsatillas are little girls. A little four-year-old boy told me in the office that "I sold my bed to my Dad, so I can sleep with Mummy." I will never forget that little smile on his face: triumphant and sweet as he had finally achieved his biggest victory. Indeed Dad slept in his bed surrounded by the teddy bears, while my Pulsatilla boy was holding Mom's hand in bed.

This refusal to grow up is easily seen at puberty when Pulsatilla is a great remedy to help the moody, insecure girl to grow up. If your teenager has been grumpy, confused, hostile and insecure since her first menstrual cycle, she needs Pulsatilla.

As Pulsatillas finally decide to grow up, though, they make excellent partners. A Pulsatilla person is not an intellectual or very cerebral person. Their prettiness and non-threatening behavior lets the husband feel strong, as if he is always in command. "You decide for us, sweetheart," she says, when it comes to going on vacation. The poor husband *thinks* he is always in control—yet upon reflection, at the end of his life, he would see that his Pulsatilla wife always got her little wish in her own subtle way.

But she brings much happiness to her husband as she does not need an exciting life. Pulsatillas adore babies, who they consider their little dolls, fussing over them and running to the doctor at the first sign of a cough. They always keep a certain childish image, easily seen in the way they dress or the way they talk to their dog or baby.

A Pulsatilla is not shy about discussing her medical history in front of people; in fact she is the first one in a homeopathy class to volunteer to come forward. And she loves group counseling, rather than a one-on-one session, as she prefers to get consolation from many people. One of my patients complained about such a woman (a Pulsatilla!) who kept interrupting a group session by constantly bursting into tears, so that everyone had to come and hug her. Twenty-some interruptions later, the sympathy of the other patients was watered down quite a bit, which Mrs. Pulsatilla could not understand.

If you succeed in giving Pulsatilla to your young Pulsatilla child, you will do yourself and your child a great favor. You will find peace of mind, since not every moment of your life will have to be dedicated to her, and she will accept attention and love in a more balanced way. Good luck!

A Pulsatilla person is likely to need these acute remedies: Children with a Pulsatilla personality are likely to come down with ailments that respond well to **Pulsatilla** acutely: ear infections, fever without thirst, hayfever. A typical Pulsatilla ear infection can be right- or left-sided, or both; acute pains starting and stopping; and a variable discharge of yellow or white pus. A little Pulsatilla girl may have a vaginal discharge that is creamy or constantly changing. (Changeability of symptoms is typical of Pulsatilla on the physical plane as are moodiness and indecisiveness on the emotional and mental planes.)

In their needy emotional state, Pulsatillas are likely to suffer from real or imaginary ailments to get attention, like the little Pulsatilla girl who complains of a tummy ache so she can stay home with mommy instead of going to school. Since Pulsatilla is a great remedy for digestive disorders, Pulsatilla will relieve her tummy ache, if it indeed exists, and in any case will help her to grow a little more independent of her mother.

Another wonderful acute remedy associated with Pulsatilla is **Kali bich.,** the un-stopper of stuffed-up noses. Remember, "If it sticks, it's Kali bich.!" referring to the thick, ropy, green, stringy mucus. **Pulsatilla** itself can be a great remedy for sinusitis and sinus headaches, especially when the sense of smell is totally gone because of stuffiness.

Natrum Muriaticum:
A Lifelong Crusader

Who is the immortal being who has never been in a Nat. mur. state of grief, loss or abandonment? Should we envy or pity that person? Envy a life with no heartbreaks or betrayals; or pity an existence that was perhaps too protected, so that life was not lived in the fullest sense.

The reasons for a grief state can start early in life and there is no way to protect against them. For instance, I had a patient whose husband was killed in an accident while she was pregnant. This immense grief *is* felt by the unborn baby, who is then born in the Nat. mur. state, which can often lead to delayed talking (or even autism, where the Nat. mur. child withdraws into his own world). Other reasons for a child going into a Nat. mur. state *intra utero* (while still in the womb) include the mother's grief at being betrayed by an unfaithful husband; separation or divorce; absence of her husband who travels all the time; and death of one of her close friends or family members.

And then there are some situations you might not think of. Any premature baby is immediately removed from the mother at birth to be put into an incubator. Certainly the baby is well taken care of—in terms of physical needs, but not emotionally.

This can lead to a Nat. mur. state.

The mother's thoughts about the pregnancy can also influence the unborn child's future personality. The unborn child is definitely aware if the mother does not want the pregnancy.

I had one patient, a man in his forties, who showed many physical symptoms which homeopaths associate with grief and abandonment. He told me he had had them his whole life, since he was born, so I knew there must have been a grief or abandonment situation while his mother was pregnant with him. He did not know of any such situation, but when he asked his mother, he found out something he never knew: his mother had decided to terminate the pregnancy and was already in the stirrups in the doctor's office, ready to have an abortion, when she changed her mind. Yet that thought stamped her unborn child to the point that he was still suffering from it forty years later.

And once the baby is born, it can suffer from grief and loss if the parents divorce, if one of them dies, or even if the parents are just too busy to care for the child properly. We call this "lack of emotional nourishment," and it can lead to a grief state just as a death in the family can.

Here is another incredible story I heard from one of my patients. She was 48 years old when she told me of a realization she had going back to her earliest days. She was the last child born into a family of seven children. She told me her mother, being exhausted (in a Sepia state!), used to put half a dozen bottles into her crib at night so she would not have to get up to feed my patient. Like a newborn in an incubator, she was taken care of food-wise, but not emotionally. It was very sad to see a full-grown woman deeply grieving this perceived abandonment from her mother nearly 50 years later.

Growing up exposes you to many more causes and triggers for a Nat. mur. state. Children can be cruel. More than once I have seen the devastation caused by rejection towards one child. Isolated and lonely, the growing child feels alone in this world, which becomes a vicious cycle that is difficult to break.

Not to mention the heartbreaks and betrayals all teenagers go through. How they cope with this is important. A Nat. mur. does not cope well with it. She tends to withdraw, wounded, isolated, and highly sensitive to further emotional hurts.

People in a Nat. mur. state suffer from a strange phenomenon. Their isolation is accentuated by the fact that they long for love, sympathy and communication, yet an inner voice forbids their acceptance and urges them to find strength within them—selves. They are like Atlas carrying the world on his shoulder, wandering around, not knowing where to deposit it. *Betrayal* is unforgivable to the

Nat. mur. person. (A Nat. mur. person can be so sensitive that she can perceive as a form of betrayal her parents lying to her about Santa Claus; one of my patients, a businessman in his thirties, mentioned this in his timeline as one of the traumas of his life!)

"Don't touch me, don't come near to me" is a strong motto. You can imagine that parents tend to feel rebuffed by the Nat. mur. child and give more affection to "easier" children—which then accentuates the loneliness of the Nat. mur. child. Often the Nat. mur. teenager expresses this loneliness with eating disorders: bulimia and anorexia often alternate in the troubled teenager. It is as though food becomes a consolation, but then causes guilt.

Every Nat. mur. is haunted by guilt feelings. "Maybe if I had stayed in the relationship longer" (when she has already stayed 10 years after it wasn't working out). "Maybe it is really my fault" (but Nat. mur. has a tendency to fall in love with the wrong partner, like a drug user or alcoholic or with an unattainable partner like a teacher or married man).

It is strange to see how this woman who is usually strong in every aspect (successful career, standing up for herself, always sympathetic for minorities and the underdog) has such a great failure rate in her relationships. Her lack of confidence is evident in her intimate relationships: she permits

163

others to take advantage of her and then bears a grudge. Nat. murs. can't let go; they remember every possible time and date where "injustice" was done to them. Many of these unfortunate Nat. mur. victims hurl themselves into some good cause like Mothers Against Drunk Drivers (a perfect way to channel the pain of losing a child).

Nat. mur.'s love for humanity is often the substitute for the love which is lacking in their own life. They become excellent psychotherapists, as they can easily feel sympathy for their unfortunate client who most likely went through the same pain as they once did. Often at this point, a Nat. mur. can give up on relationships (although they are very romantic people), and with a sharp tongue start on the reforming tour, particularly with those around her, like family members and close friends.

I have seen other dramatic Nat. mur. cases in my practice, like the case of a physician who had a legitimate rage against his partner in practice who had betrayed him. At the moment I saw him, it was already too late. He had been transformed from a brilliant person into someone who was totally withdrawn and did not communicate with his wife or anyone else. An MRI showed sudden degeneration of the brain just after this event. This should warn us to intervene with the indicated homeopathic remedies when such tragic events occur. Homeopathy was too late to save this patient.

The *withdrawal* and *retention* typical of Nat. mur. is visible on every level: she is constipated, does not urinate very often, has dry skin, hardly perspires, and suffers from premenstrual water retention, as if she wants to hold everything in. The happiest moments for most other people seem to be the most unbearable times for the Nat. mur. Holidays are sad days as they remember their deceased ones, or the relationship that went wrong, and they feel very lonely. Springtime, when we come out of our winter shell and everything blooms and takes form, can be a bad time for the closed Nat. mur. The sun only gives them headaches and painful eyes (they are very photosensitive), so they prefer the shade and always have their sunglasses on. They never feel refreshed in the morning; in fact their worst time of the day is 10 a.m. Their symptoms tend to get worse at the seashore. And they are touched by classical music but not inclined to dance: a Nat. mur. only dances with her mind, not her body (unlike a Phosphorus). Peculiar are her strong cravings for salt (Nat. mur. is prepared from salt!) and chocolate, especially premenstrually.

They come to the doctor with a minimum of information, as the physician has to earn their trust first. They are very reserved and careful people; they have been hurt too many times. Opening their deepest secret feelings to a stranger does not come easily. I had a Nat. mur. patient who covered her homeopathic questionnaire with a blank paper, as if to hide it from the outside world. I had another Nat. mur. patient who invited me to hear her sing in a recital; I was astonished at her great selection of Nat. mur. songs. A typical example was the following song:

My dear love, at least believe me, that my heart languishes without you.

Your faithful lover ever sighs.

Cruel love, put an end to this anguish.

You can see the eternal suffering, the feeling of being victimized by a cruel love, with the typical physical expression of a Nat. mur. in the acute phase: sighing. To all of us mortals for whom suffering is part of our life, never be without this wonderful remedy.

A Nat. mur. person is likely to need these acute remedies: Since someone who needs Nat. mur. is likely to suffer from water retention, **Apis** is apt to be a useful remedy for premenstrual water retention, swelling under the eyes or other forms of edema (especially around the ankles). And because her eyes are apt to be sensitive to bright light, **Bryonia** is a good bet to help her typical headaches triggered by sunlight.

To help keep her from getting into a Nat. mur. state in the first place, **Ignatia** is a wonderful remedy to give to someone suffering from acute grief, especially someone who is sighing and crying (see Ignatia in the *Guide to the Remedies*).

Sepia:
Exhausted, Dragged Down, Desperately Seeking a Vacation!

Often the source from which the remedy is taken tells us a lot about its uses. This is certainly the case for Sepia, made from the ink of the cuttlefish (also called the giant squid). The cuttlefish has the shape and form of a uterus, while Sepia is used for many disorders of the female reproductive system. The constant twitching and jerking of its head and body remind us of the Sepia patient's constant desire to move. The shades of brown and yellow which are part of the squid's astonishing camouflage system remind us of the Sepia woman's wardrobe as well as her typical pigmentation: sallow skin, a brownish mottling of the face, or the "mask of pregnancy.". The cuttlefish is a master of escape (excreting a cloud of black ink to confuse the pursuer), and escape is exactly what the Sepia woman wants when she feels totally overwhelmed. Finally, the female cuttlefish is said to have total disregard and indifference for her eggs once laid, like the exhausted Sepia woman's indifference to her family. It is also said that the male fish loses his special copulatory tentacle during intercourse—which is reflected in the depression following intercourse in the (less frequently encountered) male Sepia patient.

How does one get into a Sepia state? Many women could answer that. Typically it reflects overwork and over-responsibility. The exhaustion can easily stem from childbirth, especially if the pregnancy was hard (with Sepia being a great remedy for morning sickness), or if the delivery was difficult and/or rushed (with suction or pitocin). It is unfortunate that gynecologists don't know the power of Sepia for "postpartum blues"! Women who have had several pregnancies, miscarriages or abortions can also get into this debilitated Sepia state, drained not only of their physical energy but of their emotional energy as well. However, I have also seen women get into a Sepia state after only one pregnancy. If the baby is a screamer (a typical colicky baby) and does not want to sleep for the first three months, the mother almost inevitably will slide into this state of fatigue.

A woman in a Sepia state will say, "I am depressed" or "I am on the verge of a nervous breakdown." Indeed, she wakes up in the morning and feels there is nothing to look forward to: nothing but chores which can't wait, so overwhelming that she can't imagine being able to finish them, yet she will have to start the housework all over the next day. She never seems to get a few minutes just for herself where she can simply rest, exercise a little, read, anything to put her body and mind at peace. No wonder such a woman does not want to get out of bed. She will spend the whole day driving the kids to school and their activities, cooking, shopping, washing … the list seems endless, and by the late afternoon, she is ready to collapse. All she wants is a little nap—but this is just the moment the children come back from school, and then the "big boy," her husband, demands his dinner. He even adds insult to injury by talking about how much work he did that day (and implying that housework isn't "real work").

A Sepia woman feels pushed relentlessly with no end in sight. It is only her sense of duty that keeps her going. But there will come a time when she runs out of energy and her patience comes to an end. Trapped in her situation, feeling utterly exhausted, she tells everyone to go away and leave her alone. She will even slap her whining children without feeling a bit sorry. She is just too tired to care.

And beware of the husband asking for sex! That is just another task for her to avoid. Nor should he complain about a bad day at work. One of my patients said to her husband, "A bad day? I'll give you a bad day! I'll take out my pistols and bang! You're dead!" Another of my patients just got to the breaking point with her husband who came home from work, plopped in front of the TV and demanded that she make him a big bowl of popcorn. She took the popcorn and dumped it on his head, then got in the car and drove away for a few hours, just to be by herself—leaving her husband and kids in a panic, because they had never seen her act like this!

A Sepia woman will snap if anything extra gets added to her overloaded routine. She has to shut off or she feels she will die. She will even want to run away from this situation where she feels trapped. She may tell her husband, "You are in charge of the kids," and flee in desperation to the mall, or pack her suitcase and announce: "I am off on a little vacation and I don't want anyone coming along!"

A woman in a Sepia state may seem unsociable, but that's only because she is too tired to follow a conversation. She just wants to lie in bed with a book. Under severe stress, she may appear frozen, no longer showing emotion.

Sad to say, this Sepia state can be forced on a young girl if she has to fill her mom's shoes in the family, perhaps due to her mother's illness, absence or death. Being given so much responsibility at such a young age can mark her for the rest of her life. She may want to stay unmarried in order to avoid taking care of anyone else, or she may absolutely refuse to have children, preferring to be a successful career woman with no strings attached.

In the doctor's office she can be very critical, trying to hide the real reason of her visit: her emotional exhaustion. Often she only talks about her physical complaints, which are numerous (especially menstrual, menopausal or other hormonal symptoms).

But more often a woman in a Sepia state will burst into tears while telling her story, as crying is her only way of communicating. A Sepia will cry even more than a Pulsatilla, but her grief stems from exhaustion rather than the Pulsatilla's neediness for attention. She can have a sharp tongue; how can she feel any sympathy when she feels she can "lose it any minute"? As you can see, many women are in this unfortunate situation. I hope they will turn for help to Sepia, ready to give them a new lease on life!

A Sepia woman is likely to need these acute remedies:
The main thing a woman in a Sepia state needs is help from a homeopath, who can prescribe remedies in the right professional potencies. She can also benefit by using **Sepia** acutely in situations such as these:

Many women, and especially women in a Sepia state, are likely to need Sepia for dysmenorrhea (with the typical Sepia symptom of a bearing-down feeling in the uterus, as though it might slide out through the vagina!) Sepia is also good for morning sickness, vomiting during pregnancy, and hot flashes during menopause. It can also be used acutely for PMS symptoms such as irritability, weepiness and depression. I often tell my women patients to protect themselves against exhaustion during the Thanksgiving-Christmas season by taking Sepia 200C (3 pellets, dry in the mouth, as needed).

"Readers of his books rave about his ability to teach them about medicine as well as health and well-being."
—*Napa Trade Journa*

Human Condition: Critical
An introduction to homeopathy

The perfect companion to **The People's Repertory,** this book provides a more in-depth explanation of what homeopathy is and how it works, emphasizing chronic illnesses. Dr. Luc explains the pillars of good health and the true causes of chronic diseases such as Chronic Fatigue Syndrome. He describes the multiple factors causing such diseases to become widespread in our civilization, while explaining homeopathy's powerful tools to combat them. Dr. Luc helps the reader to discover and heal neglected emotional factors affecting his health. For a thorough and easy-to-understand introduction to the laws and concepts of homeopathy, there is no better book than **Human Condition: Critical.** This book won second prize among 3800 papers at the First World Congress of Traditional Medicine.

216 pages, $12.95

Human Condition: Critical *is a very readable and interesting explanation of homeopathy and its ability to treat* *emotional factors in disease. It provides knowledge necessary for people to make informed choices about practitioners, the healing process, and the use of this effective and inexpensive form of medicine."*

—Townsend Letter for Doctors

"Renowned physician, acupuncturist and homeopath Dr. De Schepper urges his readers to take medical matters into their own hands. Homeopathy is made accessible and fascinating by his easy writing style and manageable, yet comprehensive, wealth of knowledge. This worthy book is easy to pick up and hard to put down."

—Napa Trade Journal

"The author has been thoroughly schooled in Western medicine, homeopathy and acupuncture, giving him a much broader view of health than most doctors. Here he draws social attention to the environmental causes of ailments, stressing that it is only by addressing these causes, and not merely the symptoms of disease, that we can ever hope to bring about a cure."

—Bookpeople

What About Men?

How can women avoid getting involved and obsessed with men—men who are clearly wrong for them, who are abusive, addictive, too complacent, procrastinators, not exciting enough, or full of anxieties. Using his extensive training in Western medicine, acupuncture and homeopathy, Dr. Luc has, for the first time, written a book that gives almost scientific clues to getting to know a man and choosing the right one for you. This book gives you emotional and mental portraits as well as the characteristic physical symptoms that you can look for in men.

These portraits are like the ones in **The People's Repertory,** but are specifically geared to men, and they incorporate the wisdom of Traditional Chinese Medicine as well as homeopathy. They will help you to predict whether a man is likely to control you, stimulate you or be chaotic for you before the damage is done. A questionnaire helps you determine what kind of man you have in your life in all his many facets.

This is not only a book for women. Men will read about their weaknesses and be able to correct them with homeopathic remedies before they are transformed into real diseases. When you read this book, you may cry, smile, or laugh ... but you will never look at a man the same way!

244 pages, $12.95

Full of Life: How to Achieve and Maintain Peak Immunity

Full of Life describes a complete program for achiev-- ing and maintaining peak immunity, from a doctor who has cured thousands of patients suffering from CFIDS (Chronic Fatigue and Immune Dysfunction Syndrome). It contains a formula of holistic and nu- tritional healing methods and gives readers a chance to regain their strength and renew their lives. You will take a self-scoring questionnaire to see if you are at risk for immune-suppressed conditions. If you suspect that you are suffering from CFIDS, viral or yeast infections, *Full of Life* gives you specific tools for working with your doctor. You can become an active participant in the diagnosis and treatment of your condition.

The common sense approach of the book does away with the many unproven viral theories as it focuses on real causes leading to a decline in your immune system. By recognizing and correcting these causes immediately, you will have instant clues to follow a highly effective program for both preventing immune system breakdown, and healing it once it's happened.

222 pages, $12.95

"Dr. Luc De Schepper, one of this country's foremost holistic practitioners, has written a sensitive, positively-oriented book which clearly explains the conditions that have developed in this world to create our current epidemics of CFIDS and AIDS. This book serves to educate the reader on all the nutritional and holistic approaches to these illnesses and does so with compassion and a positive outlook."

—To Your Health, NY

"*Full of Life* is a very informative book for the lay person, on a subject that has been given short shrift. It goes a long way to educating health consumers to the benefits of preventive medicine, as well as alerting them to the importance of protecting their first line of defense against illness."

—Townsend Letter for Doctors

"One of the best books around on CFIDS, AIDS and immuno-suppressed conditions from a leading medical expert. A vital, honest look into the heart of the 20th century's most pressing problems."

—The Book Reader,
America's most independent review of new books

Candida: The Symptoms, the Causes, the Cure

Candida, commonly known as a yeast infection, is increasing at an alarming rate. If you or members of your family have headaches, poor memory, allergies, gas, constipation, depression, and/or loss of libido and don't know why, you may be among the one out of three people presently suffering from this condition.

The overuse of antibiotics, cortisone and "the pill," combined with refined and preserved foods have made Candida more prevalent than ever. Yeasts, stress, nutritional deficiencies, sugar consumption, air pollution, hormone imbalance, toxins and vitamin deficiencies can also cause Candida.

This book—by a doctor who has successfully treated thousands of patients with Candida—contains new medical discoveries that could change your life. The symptoms of this disease and step-by-step therapy are described. Chapters dealing with the psychological profile of how to cope with the disease, provide the patient and the family with the necessary tools for help and understanding, from the onset to the cure of this condition. Abundant recipes and answers to the most frequently-asked questions are included.

150 pages, $10.00

"The solution to an irritating and debilitating problem is contained in this practical and easy-to-follow guide to good health. And the recipes for healthy eating are quite delicious too!"

—**Foulsham Publisher**, London, England

*"**Candida** by Luc De Schepper is the newest book on this subject and yes—it's also the best. The author is extremely thorough, yet so easy to understand that the book is a pleasure to read. Every section of **Candida** is pertinent and interesting."*

—**Alive Books**, Canada

"An extremely interesting examination of the widely different problems that can arise from invasion of the human system by the common yeast."

—**Health World,** CA

"Written by a practicing MD, acupuncturist and homeopath, the author has made a thorough presentation of this topic, providing great detail in his proposal for therapy."

—**Red Wing**, MA

How to Dine Like the Devil and Feel Like a Saint: Goodbye to Guilty Eating

This is a complete diet book that promotes well-being and health. What sets it apart from any other diet book is the explanation of the "three diet phases," *cleansing, stabilizing, and Full of Life* phase with a 28-day, easy-to-follow recipe program. A chapter entitled "Life on the Road" teaches you how to maintain a healthy life-style when entering the restaurant world. It offers key profiles of foods like quinoa, amaranth and other ancient grains. And it contains clear, easy- to-follow recipes to prepare healthy salads, dressings, biscuits, muffins, breads, and—let's not forget—*"Party items!"* A book that is a must for every kitchen!

222 pages, $17.95

"In his mission to teach others how to attain and maintain health, Dr. De Schepper presents dietary factors that preserve health. How to Dine like the Devil is full of useful information; and it encourages people to take control of their own well-being."

—Townsend Letter for Doctors

"A book of delicious recipes and friendly advice including the seven principles of healthy eating. Dr. De Schepper pays special attention to those occasions when it is more difficult to stick to wise eating habits—when there is no time (or energy) to make a decent meal and during holidays and special occasions." **—Bookpeople**, CA

Musculoskeletal Diseases and Homeopathy

This book is the first one on homeopathic applications to musculoskeletal diseases. It is very clinically oriented and therefore a must for every chiropractor, medical doctor, osteopath and acupuncturist who wants to incorporate homeopathy. It can be used by the physician who has a budding interest in the topic, as well as by the advanced homeopathic physician.

Organized in three sections, *Musculoskeletal Diseases* deals first with homeopathic philosophy, principles and laws; what potencies to use; mistakes in prescribing; homeopathic case taking; management of the patient; and the role of palliation in incurable diseases. Part Two discusses the most frequent encountered clinical conditions, including a definition, etiology, symptomatology, Western medical approach, prognosis, and the different homeopathic remedies according to their value for each condition. Part Three consists of the Materia Medica of the same remedies used in Part Two in such a way that they can be easily remembered.,

Because of its easy organization, the book comes in handy at any given moment during the consultation. A quick differential diagnosis can be made by the physician. And because of its very important first part, the physician will always be able to manage the patient's case on further visits.

200 pages, $39.95

Acupuncture in Practice

What sets this book apart from other textbooks is its thoroughly clinical approach. It is practice-oriented, teaching step-by-step how to diagnose and treat the patient, therefore making it a must for every acupuncturist, whether beginning or advanced. It can also be used by the physician, osteopath or chiropractor who has a budding interest in the topic. Organized in two sections, the book deals first with acupuncture principles and laws, the concept of Qi, Yin and Yang, the Five Elements, the different channels and their applications, Chinese diagnostics with pulse and tongue picture, the theory of Tsang-Fu, the Eight Conditions, the most opportune moment to treat, Tchong Mo, Moxibustion and a dialectic of the acupuncture points.

Part two discusses frequently encountered clinical conditions with their acupuncture interpretation and treatment plan. It contains chapters about rheumatoid diseases, diseases of the blood, psychological diseases, pregnancy and delivery, impotence and sterility, menopause, tinnitus and deafness, endometriosis, perspiration, modern diseases like chronic fatigue (CFIDS) and the Gulf War Syndrome, and how to treat and approach complicated patient cases. Also discussed are the clinically important Sky-Window and Barrier points. Numerous drawings and clinical examples serve to clarify each subject under discussion.   202 pages, $39.95

ORDER FORM

copy this order form and mail it with a check or money order to:

Full of Life Publishing
P.O. Box 31025
Santa Fe, NM 87594

Quantity	Title	Total
___	*The People's Repertory* @ $9.95	_____
___	*Human Condition Critical* @ $12.95	_____
___	*What About Men?* @ $12.95	_____
___	*Full of Life* @ $12.95	_____
___	*Candida: the Symptoms, the Causes, the Cure* @ $10.00	_____
___	*How to Dine Like the Devil* @ $17.95	_____
___	*Musculoskeletal Diseases and Homeopathy* @ $39.95	_____
___	*Acupuncture in Practice* @ $39.95	_____

Subtotal _____

New Mexico residents add 6.5% sales tax _____

Shipping: $3.00 first book,
$1.00 each additional _____

TOTAL _____

Dr. Luc De Schepper is the founder of the New School of Homeopathy for health care professionals in Cambridge, Mass. and the author of ten books on homeopathy, acupuncture and holistic health care. He recently retired from private practice as a homeopathic family physician in order to devote himself full time to teaching and writing about homeopathy. Previously Dr. Luc was in private practice in preventive medicine, homeopathy and acupuncture in Santa Monica, CA, where he became nationally known for his success in treating candida and chronic fatigue.

Dr. Luc has medical licenses in Belgium and the United States; acupuncture licenses in Holland and California; and a Ph.D. in acupuncture (with related studies in homeopathy) from the International Society of Acupuncture in Paris. He has received the Diploma of the British Institute of Homeopathy (D.I. Hom.) as well as the Certificate of the Hahnemann Academy of North America (C.Hom.). Dr. Luc has appeared on numerous television shows in the United States and abroad as well as being interviewed on dozens of radio shows. He is fluent in four languages and is a popular lecturer in the fields of acupuncture and homeopathy.

Health care practitioners interested in studying homeopathy with Dr. Luc are encouraged to visit the New School of Homeopathy's website at www.LMhomeopathy.com or to write to the school at 5A Lancaster St., Cambridge, MA 02140 for information and application materials.